Dead Man on a Bike

Dead Man on a Bike

Riding with Cancer

by Wayne Tefs

TURNSTONE PRESS

Turnstone Press
Artspace Building
206-100 Arthur Street
Winnipeg, MB
R3B 1H3 Canada
www.TurnstonePress.com

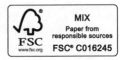

Turnstone Press gratefully acknowledges the assistance of the Canada Council
for the Arts, the Manitoba Arts Council, the Government of Canada through
the Canada Book Fund, and the Province of Manitoba through the Book Pub-
lishing Tax Credit and the Book Publisher Marketing Assistance Program.

Quotations by Charles M. Schulz (5) and James E. Starrs (103) are used with
permission.

Printed and bound in Canada by Friesens for Turnstone Press.

Library and Archives Canada Cataloguing in Publication

Tefs, Wayne, 1947-, author
    Dead man on a bike : riding with cancer / Wayne Tefs.

ISBN 978-0-88801-529-7 (pbk.)

    1. Tefs, Wayne, 1947- --Health. 2. Cancer--Patients--Canada--
Biography. 3. Cyclists--Canada--Biography. 4. Cycling--Therapeutic
use. 5. Authors, Canadian (English)--20th century--Biography. I. Title.

PS8589.E37Z53 2016   C813'.54   C2014-907892-7 *for Kristen*

Dead Man on a Bike

When the spirits are low, when the day appears dark, when work becomes monotonous, when hope hardly seems worth having, just mount a bicycle and go out for a spin down the road, without thought on anything but the ride you are taking.
~ Arthur Conan Doyle

J ust past Honey Bee Park the road rises slightly and DMB stands up on the pedals to maintain speed. On one side of the road a sprawling housing development, on the other open desert, spreading to the base of the Catalina Mountains. The sun beats down on the tarmac. The mountains in the distance are more sharply outlined than usual: it rained during the night, settling the desert dust of Tucson. The morning air is fresh, there's a breeze from the east, noticeable at the top of the crest he's just crossing over. When he gets there, he gasps for breath; the big tumour in his liver pinches up his belly button; he inhales deeply. This is not hard cycling, but it's hard work for him. He's a dead man cycling, he's the Dead Man on a Bike.

Here the road begins to descend. The tires whirr, the air rushing past ruffles the collar of his cycling jersey. Forty kilometres an hour, fifty. The blacktop is smooth, the bike lane wide and happily free of grit and gravel and little objects thrown from the wheels of cars: *bagwell*. The bike is swooping downhill. DMB's heart thumps in his throat. This is what he came out to do.

This is the fun of riding a bike: the abandon of letting it go, of moving hands into the drops, crouching into the tuck position, head down, knees pressed against the top tube, elbows in, maximum aerodynamics. Fifty-five k.p.h. The road sweeps in long curves, straightens over a gulch bridge—*washes* they're called in Arizona. Thumpty thumpty thumpty over the bridge. DMB's view of the road joggles. The tarmac is a blur of black rumples. The road plunges some twenty or so metres, then flattens. Wheeee. The bike bounces over ripples in the tarmac as it nears the bottom, there's a moment when control of the machine rushes precariously to the edge of disaster, he feels the wheels hit sand and begin to slide away under him, DMB's going down, water bottle bouncing free of the cage, helmet rolling one way, energy bars another, the bike skidding to the curbing, DMB's body scraping and cracking on the tarmac: *yard sale,* cyclists say.

But he's okay. The wheels stay under. To be a cyclist he thinks is to be slightly mad, to intentionally blind oneself to the prospect of death. But that's what it's all about. Yes. Once again he's defied the odds, once again he's ridden the knife edge of mayhem and come out on the other side, heart flailing with the certitude of life. He's alive under the desert sun. The tires whirr. A dog in the housing development barks repeatedly, yap yap yap; they pick up the high pitch of the wheels' spokes. It drives them crazy.

Suddenly across the tarmac in front of the bike a tiny black scuttle—vole? What you doing out past sunrise, little buddy, with hawks sitting atop telephone poles and riding air currents up and down? Scoot, vole, find your tiny hole in the desert sand, dig in, hunker in a safe spot under a dusty sage bush. Life is on the line out here.

The surface rises slightly as DMB approaches Tangerine Road. The bike slows as he comes up to the red light at the intersection. He brakes, kicks one cleat out of the pedal and brings the machine to a stop. Slowly the roaring in his ears stops. Arms no longer atremble. A guy in a car beside him, elbow propped on the window ledge, cigarette dangling between two fingers says to him, chuckling and nodding his head: "That's the way, Dude, bring it on!"

Life is like a ten-speed bicycle; most of us have gears we never use.
~ Charles M. Schulz

One of my earliest memories is of standing in the kitchen of our house on Sherbrook Street with blood pouring down my three-year-old face. My tricycle had bashed into the wall of an apartment block a stone's throw away and my skull had come into collision with those sturdy red bricks that buildings were made of in the era between the wars. Abrasive to the touch and sharp-edged. Blood was dripping off my chin onto my shoes. My mother was fussing around with towels and commiseration. Blubbing, and aware of the concern on my mother's face, and also thinking I'd done something dreadful, I claimed someone had pushed me, and years later, my older sister, in a fit of guilt, seemed prepared to accept responsibility; but it's as likely I drove into the wall on my own, but was reluctant to confess that to my mother. Like most males, I've always been prone to stick my hand into the wood-chipper *just to see*. In any case, my mother stanched the flow of blood and cleaned up my face, and though "stitches" were spoken of, the bandage she applied appeared to preclude the visit to the hospital and within hours all was well, though there was no more riding on that day.

It was my first "crash," and a memorable one. Though it was by no means the last. Had I been aware of such things, I might have noted it was the initial incident in my life where cycling and life-threatening jeopardy crossed into each other.

The tricycle was undamaged: one of those red and white steel units, forged from one solid ingot, it seemed, and able to withstand the endless abuses and goof-ups of children. What would it have taken to damage it? Perhaps the wheels of one of the delivery trucks that blundered up and down the back lanes in those days, delivering coal or heating oil, huffing and chuffing diesel. Though you wouldn't have staked money on that. Those trikes were indestructible.

When my father came home from the service station he owned and operated at the corner of Sherbrook and Ellice, he learned of the day's momentous occurrence and briefly examined the bandage on my head. He asked, "How long was the cut open to the air?" My mother was quizzical. She told him: about five minutes. "Good thing it wasn't longer," he said, nodding around the smoke issuing from his pipe; "no knowing how many brains may have leaked out if it had been longer." I started to wonder about that, touching the bandage with my fingertips tentatively; I wasn't sure how many I might have had to spare; I was no match for my older sister, that I knew. But before my ruminations came to grief, my mother shushed him and he winked at me and patted me on the shoulder, so I knew there was nothing to worry about. I'd have enough brains to get by on, it seemed. He did not offer anything more; hugging and shows of affection were not in the armoury of the men who took off uniforms in 1945 after their term of service. They'd been educated in the school of hard knocks, where a wink or a brief pat on the shoulder passed for acknowledgment, and tenderness was not in the arsenal at all.

As a boy a decade later I had a paper route in the mining town where my sisters and I spent our formative years, and I delivered the *Winnipeg Free Press*, one day late on a hefty old clunker that my parents had bought me, or that had been passed down from someone no longer needing it. I bounced around the roads of Atikokan on it with two brothers who were the sons of our church minister. They had new matching blue bikes, memorable for the sweep of their handlebars, like the appendages of long-horn cattle, and fat balloon-like tires. We cruised the town's roads on our travels between our respective households, Neil and Lee and

I. And I dreamed of the day when my savings from the paper route would secure me such a magnificent machine. I was counting the dollars in my bank account, it seemed, forever—which was probably one summer—before the price of the bike was within reach. It was a CCM, perhaps named "roadster" or some such thing, and it came from Winnipeg by way of Eaton's store, where it had been ordered from the catalogue. It was everything a boy of twelve in 1958 could dream of: sweeping lines, big tires, bright red and white enamel paint that gleamed in the summer sun—just like the tricycle, come to think of it.

My bike was the envy of the neighbourhood for about three weeks. Lee and Neil and my best pal, Johnny, were among those who got to take a test ride. Others had to stand on the sidelines waving pompoms of envy, appraising the bike and wondering how they might acquire one. Then two brothers from Alabama moved in several doors down from ours and envy of my wheels was overshadowed by curiosity and delight in the Brennans' accents. The two brothers were tall and beefy, nice enough fellows, but not of our ilk. The older was already attending military school in the US, and his younger brother, who was our age, was scheduled to follow in his footsteps come the autumn. Still, those accents. I remember calling on Mrs. Brennan to ask whether she wanted a subscription to the *Free Press*, a dubious ruse; I was there to hear her voice. "Whye, it is mighty kind of ya'll to offer," she drawled, "but I doan belleeve we will be re-choirin' that pah-tic-alar ayetem of infomashun," sweet as syrup, and I almost peed my pants.

We swooped up and down the hills on our bikes, the Sanders boys and me. And Johnny joined us, or just he and I haunted the streets when the Sanders boys were otherwise engaged. Johnny was shorter than me and more athletic in the gymnastic way. We were both fans of The Lone Ranger, who, impressively to our pre-pubescent imaginations, could snatch up his fallen Stetson from a galloping horse when it got knocked off in an encounter with villains. We threw our caps on the sandy square that served as the base of the hockey rink in winter and set out to emulate the masked avenger, with accompanying cries of *ke-mo sah-bee*, which I believe we thought might have meant something akin to *Geronimo!* Whisking up our caps became something of an obsession between us for most of one summer. Johnny could almost accomplish the feat, his fingertips just dandling the cloth of his cap, but all I ever managed was to drive over my cap and then collapse into the sand as it slowed the bike's progress, my legs and arms entangled in my magnificent red and white CCM, sand running into my sneakers, and my hips and shoulders banged up from falls.

I loved riding that bike. Being on the move. Motion in and of itself fascinates and captivates the young, a holdover, likely, from the days not so recently past when as toddlers we were learning the joys of walking and running, being free of the dual constraints of crawling and our parents picking us up and plunking us down at *their* whim. That ecstatic freedom carried over, for me, at least, into bicycle riding. My schoolmates too. We zipped around the roads of town with abandon, and ventured out of town, too, on the blacktop stretches that ran to the mines and the logging camps nearby, and even the one highway out of town, the highway to what was then known as The Lakehead. Some of my pals were daredevils, doing tricks like wheelies and riding backwards on the saddle, long before this became standard practice among the BMX generations. I was not of that type. I enjoyed zipping along the blacktop roads that snaked through and around town. Atikokan was the site of two iron mines in the Canadian Shield, and the terrain was quite hilly, so there were plenty of undulating streets with long, sweeping curves, and I loved the freedom of swooping down the blacktop at high speed, wind in hair, the bicycle half out of control. I rode often with my pals, but equally often I rode alone, revelling in the quasi-loneliness of being by myself on the road, separate and untrammelled, half lost in the dream-like state that comes so easily on a bicycle. I was experiencing for the first time the heady brew of latitude and abandon and vulnerability that comes with a bicycle. I was exploring what it meant to be a Self. And my shiny red and white CCM opened the door onto the risk-taking that has fuelled and dogged my adulthood.

Whatever became of that bike? The iron mines at Atikokan—Steep Rock and Caland—experienced a dramatic downturn in the early '60s; my father's business went bankrupt; we moved to Fort Frances, where he started another business, and then to Steinbach, where he tried again, and finally back to Winnipeg, where he settled in as a house builder and supported his family as men of his generation did, tirelessly and uncomplainingly, the way they had learned to do in the army. The CCM went missing in action somewhere along the line, and it was more than twenty years before I owned another bicycle.

DEAD MAN ON A BIKE

Life is like riding a bicycle—in order to keep your balance,
you must keep moving.
~ Albert Einstein

It is the summer of 2014 and DMB is out on the bicycle. He doesn't know how many more rides there might be. A heart attack in March surprised him, the doctors, everyone; unrelated to the cancer, but not without effect on it.

He rides beside Kristen, who has slowed to his pace, tries not to show worry in her face. He wears long sleeves in spite of the warm day—he's always cold now, and so very very thin. He turns the pedals, flat pedals so he doesn't have to negotiate with the cleats, isn't locked into his bike. Since the heart attack his balance betrays him, he has to be ready to drop a foot, catch the ground with a toe, right himself before crashing. He changed the pedals last week, after falling from a near stand-still when he couldn't de-cleat in time. He didn't tell Kristen about the fall.

She has taken the day off work today. More and more often she works from home, she says to keep him company, but he knows she's started to worry. Twenty years of battling cancer, twenty years to face that challenge, only to be brought up short by a heart attack. The cardio-oncologist said, "There are four ways a man can die: cancer, heart attack, stroke, or getting hit by a car. You should stay off the road, my friend."

He pushes the pedals, up, down.

They have decided to ride to the Vietnamese restaurant for lunch. It is one of the few places he can still enjoy. The food is tasty, and he's able to eat most of what is served him. They wait at the light, crossing busy Pembina Highway on foot, rolling the bikes. He pushes his pace, and barely crosses before the light turns. He sighs. Gone are the days of negotiating three or four lanes of busy roadway, signalling through roundabouts with a quick flick of the arm. They remount and pedal slowly along the chopped-up sidewalk to the restaurant.

After a good meal they retrace their steps and mount the bikes on a quiet neighbourhood street. After lunch, he is even slower, and hangs his head. When he looks up again, DMB sees Kristen has pulled ahead. Panic fills his throat, the kind of panic he hasn't felt since being a kid on the school ground, the bell ringing, everyone charging ahead: "Hey, wait up, wait for me!" Don't leave me behind, he thinks, just as she turns her head, looks back, slows to a stop. DMB is being left behind, whether he likes it or not. It can't be much longer, now.

He shakes his head, pushes the thought aside, rides up beside Kristen, who turns a pedal, picks up pace beside him and smiles ruefully. "Sorry," she says, "I got lost in thought." He shakes his head—no worries—and together they ride home.

I bought it on Queen Street in Toronto, that first genuine adult machine, in the basement of a shop where the proprietor pointed me when I inquired about used bicycles. It was white and it caught my eye because it had black bar tape and a tiny maple leaf stamped on the down tube. It was a Peugeot, the famous French brand ridden by numerous winners of Le Tour and other big-name races, though this bicycle was manufactured in Quebec, I later learned; hence the maple leaf. It was just a bit small for me but I put down my $100 and rode back to the apartment where I was living on Avenue Road near Eglinton, sweating up the hills under the summer sun in jeans and a long-sleeve shirt, a mistake I promised myself to never make again.

I was in my late thirties, on leave from my teaching post in Winnipeg, taking a sabbatical and writing a book. It was an idyllic life, complemented by the bicycle. I passed my days writing, reading at the Robarts Library at the University of Toronto, where I was an alumnus, and playing tennis with my college pal, Peter. Before buying the Peugeot, I'd been employing the public transit system and doing a lot of walking. The bicycle gave me freedom to ride to the tennis courts where we played; to make quick trips to the grocery store and coffee shop; to travel at my own whim, rather than the timetable of the transit system; to explore side streets and byways I would never otherwise have investigated. From its inception as a commuter vehicle, the bicycle has served this worthy purpose—and many others. It was a vital player in the suffragette movement of the late nineteenth and early twentieth centuries, allowing women, especially young women, to escape the restraints of their homes and meet each other (and men) away from the scalding eyes of their parents.

That liberty is at the core of every cycling moment: whether it's the roadies scooting along the Chiantigiana on Sunday mornings in their neon jerseys, or the retired school mistress in my neighbourhood pedalling her ancient touring machine with its front basket holding her pet rabbit, or the wild men on their mountain bikes at the "rampage" challenge, plummeting down dusty, ochre canyons in Utah. The bicycle opens a window onto adventure. It may be a quest, it may be a voyage, it may be a challenge; it is always a letting go of the old self and putting on of the new. You cannot discount the role that *thrill* plays in any bike ride. Part of the allure is the sheer peril of cycling: the chances of the crash. On two wheels you're always only a moment away from falling. It's a high risk/high reward activity. You gain a sense of life by putting your life on the line.

The Peugeot was a "racer," with a double chain ring and a rear cluster of gears that gave its rider ten gears to manoeuvre through, depending on terrain, a "ten speed." I did not ride it that way. For me it was a commuter bike, my transport around the university and about the city, and it mainly stayed in one gear. It served me well in that capacity, reliable, manoeuvrable, and I brought it back to Winnipeg when I returned to my teaching post the following autumn. There I rode it differently in the summers following my return, clicking through the gears on sunny days on ten- and fifteen-kilometre jaunts around my neighbourhood and on city streets connecting one neighbourhood to another. Writing is an avocation that's mostly headwork, and getting out on the bike provided a welcome break from thinking and sitting in front of a computer screen, a physical oasis in an otherwise dry mental landscape. The Peugeot had racing handlebars, a tiny, hard saddle, and all the other features of the standard racing bike of its day: twenty-five-millimetre tires, toe clips, water bottle cages; and a slick derailleur system. I rode it hard and fast, hair flying off my collar in the style of Guy Lafleur, helmetless on the road, as he had been on the ice. Fortunately, I did not crash and crack my skull, the triumph of good luck over flawed judgment.

I had entered the world of road cycling, where freedom dwells, where the buzz beckons, where all is promised and much hazarded.

The Peugeot was my ride through the late '80s and early '90s, good transport, a hardy road machine that was not elegant but was durable. I would have been happy to bang around on it for years, but in the early '90s I met my current wife, Kristen, and though she had a road bike, she preferred off-road riding, so we bought a couple of entry-level mountain bikes, Trek Antelopes, both blue in colour, with twenty-eight-inch wheels and twist-style shifters on the handlebars, the newest thing.

On a Saturday afternoon we set off from her parents' place near Headingley, headed for the part of Beaudry Park on the north side of the river. The ride took us through agricultural fields to the east, in the direction of the Headingley Jail. There was a hard-packed gumbo road several hundred metres distant that ran north/south into the park where there were cycling trails, and that road was our objective. At first the riding was easy, skirting a fallow field by way of a grassy border; but soon the grasses bordering the field grew ankle- and then knee-deep—home, it turned out, to various kinds of jumping insects, flies, and mosquitoes—and when we sought an easier course through the ploughed field, it turned out to be corrugated gumbo. From the grass verge it had looked dry and hard but depressions in the terrain were, closer up, quagmires of standing and stagnant water, bogs measuring several metres across. In no time the wheels of the shiny new bikes were clogged with mud, and we were sweating to keep them upright, fly-bitten, our arms, wrists and legs screaming NO! So this was off-road riding: taxing, unpredictable, likely to end up in a crash or with us leaping from the saddle to jerk around marshes, rock piles, sloughs, sandlots, busted-up blacktop, all of which awaited in the following weeks as we put the bikes—and ourselves—to the test in the Sandilands and the margins of Birds Hill Park and the rough tracks near Lac du Bonnet. The Antelopes took it all in stride: they were heavy, robust, and clumsy, but if you had the stamina and determination to keep the pedals turning, they got you there, *puff-puff, pass the water bottle.* An exercise in endurance, but even given that, a cartload of fun. We pushed ourselves on those bikes, enjoying what little speed we could develop on downhills and perilous descents over rocks, and ruts, and tree branches. We ground to a halt often, and fell, and we leapt off and let the bikes go on a few of those descents, clattering ahead of us over stones and boulders, and through tangled underbrush. Soon they were scraped and scratched and a little worse for wear—as were we.

We took them to the Eastern Townships and the Madeleine Islands, and shipped them to England where we did a tour of the Cotswolds.

Limestone. Limestone cliffs, walls, roads, dust. Half golden, honey-coloured limestone; in the slanting light of afternoon you pass a low stone wall, backgrounded by green rolling hills; you sense this gently undulating landscape of shrubs, yew trees and white sheep could be "God's country," which is what "Cotswolds" means, they say. Lovely riding, too: winding country lanes, quiet side roads, pretty villages right out of *Britain Magazine.* Chief among them: Stratford.

We roll out on the mountain bikes on a sunny morning on what is to be a "fine" day, which in England means warmish with a lesser likelihood of rain. We're heading first to an ox drove, what once was a hard-packed track along a ridge, frequented by merchants, farmers, and travellers as the connecting link between villages, the tracks in the valleys below susceptible to England's soggy weather, likely to be impassable mud on most days.

On the ridge proper the work is hard. Up a rise at 15 kph, then down a descent at 30 kph. The big tires of the mountain bike bounce over the track. The view of the path in front jiggles along with the jouncing of the bike. Wrists ache, the small of the back takes every jolt in the track. Bees buzz around when you slow. Overhead hawks swoop and glide. There's no one else on the ridge. At the eight-kilometre point of the ride there's a pheasant on the track, its red and black head bobbing as it pecks in the gravel verge. For the briefest of seconds Kristen risks lifting one hand off the handlebars to point. I nod. When the bikes approach, the pheasant whirls up in a flurry of feathers and wing strokes, a magnificent display of reds, oranges, blacks, greys, and a sound like a drum beating. It passes directly over our heads and then turns into the bushes that run along the ox drove, and then the fields beyond.

We stop for water. The terrain is too rutted and rough to hazard drinking on the bicycles, to hazard one hand on the handlebars. Purple flowers grow on a low bush. Wasps buzz about. We snap a photo. At 11:00 the sun is high and on the sheltered ridge path it's hot. Our mouths are dry. We grin. Our heart monitors tell us we're close to the red zone. This is what we came to do. Back on the bikes we pass a disused quarry and skirt a wood. Here the ridge rises, the grade is becoming steeper, the rear wheels slip in the gravel and spin on the hard-packed mud. We're breathing hard, fingers clenched on the bars, legs pumping to keep the machines moving. Better to stand or stay seated? Up, up, the pitch is challenging, then it's gruelling, we're in low gears and then granny gear. We're doing the ascent to Broadway Tower, one of the highest points in the Cotswolds, 1083 feet above sea level and a 600-foot climb from the base where we began only minutes ago.

We get to the top, hearts hammering and sweat running into our eyes. There's a parking lot to one side and two cars are parked facing each other, their drivers, men in their early thirties, are talking through rolled-down windows. Cigarettes smouldering in their hands. One of them looks at us and smiles. We've slowed and are wiping our foreheads with the backs of our hands. "Doing it the energetic way, are you?" one quips. They both smile. We hop off the bicycles and pause for a moment, palms on knees, the bikes resting against a fence. "Yikes," I say between gasps of breath. The men laugh and shake their heads. "Good on ya," the guy says.

After a moment his mate asks, "Where you from, then?"

"Canada," Kristen says.

The guy says, "Alfie here, his da moved to Edmonton."

"Edmonton," I say. "It's like the city we come from. Winnipeg?"

The guys look at each other and shake their heads. "We hope to get to Manchester one day," Alfie says, laughing. "See the Little Red Devils at Old Trafford."

"Not world travellers, us," his mate adds. At first I think he means the two of them, but then it occurs to me he might mean folks from around here, maybe all Britons. Which would be surprising for a country that once had an Empire. In school in the '50s a big map hung over the blackboard, sponsored by Nielsen's chocolates: it showed all the countries of the world, the British Empire in pink. Empire. Along with "Oh, Canada" and "The Maple Leaf Forever," we kids named Podolski and Zahn, Zeufiele and Beuchler, living in a remote mining town in the north of Ontario, learned to sing (with gusto!) "Rule Britannia": "Rule Britannia, Britannia rules the waves …"

Back on the bikes, we climb over rocks, sweating to keep them upright, and then meander along a mud path through a field of black-nosed sheep. On their butts have been splotched plate-sized circles of blue dye. They eye us nervously, crowd together at our approach, and scuttle away when we pass. We dismount to go through a metal fence, the gate creaks as it swings open. A metal sign is attached to the clasp: KEEP CLOSED. Then it's uphill again, over boulders, slip-sliding, gearing down. The track curves around a wood at the crest of a hill, then drops through clots of cow pats and transforms into gravel. Ahead of us we can see for several kilometres. A group of hikers is rounding a curve on the track we're following in the distance, bright backpacks slung over shoulders, white T-shirts, hats bobbing. They too are making for Snowshill, which can be seen in the valley before us, a cluster of stone buildings, a church steeple, the glint of car hoods.

We chuckle over the West country town names: Stow-on-the Wold, Hook Norton, Tally Ho, Upper and Lower Slaughter, Temple Guiting, Birdlip, Dumbleton, Chew Magna, Chipping Campden, Great Tew, Wooten Bassett, Gorsley Common, Odbury on the Hill, Nether Wallop, and Snig's End. We're heading to Snowshill (pronounced "snozzle") where we'll stop for lunch.

At the Snowshill Arms I order grilled trout on a bed of rice with beets and peas to one side, and Kristen has a wedge of Stilton cheese accompanied by a pickled onion, two slabs of bread with butter and carrot sticks. Washed down with pints of local ale and bitter. The ramblers we encountered on the rough bridleway on our descent from Broadway Tower have arrived and they carry their pints and plates onto the grassy square across from the pub proper. They put their backpacks at their feet. There are benches but most sit on the grass and admire the blocky but beautiful

Norman church inside a well-preserved limestone fence. Within the little yard two towering yew trees throw shade over the cemetery surrounding the church and its ménage of ancient, tilting, and indecipherable tombstones. Crimson and amarillo flowers in narrow beds front the main entrance. Picture postcard stuff.

A pair of the hikers sits besides us. Doris says, "We're doing the Cotswold Way. Fifty miles we've done, with another fifty or so to go. Not in one day." She laughs. Her accent is south of London. "About ten miles a day."

"Lovely inns," Albert adds. They're a retired couple, white hair, paunches, red faces.

I ask, "Good weather?"

"Fine," Doris.

"A treat," Albert says.

"We had a run-in with a bull in a field yesterday," Doris says. "Scared us some."

Albert laughs. "We were scampering for the fence, that's for certain."

I say, "It's an arranged tour, like, with a guide and a route and so on?"

"Terry," Albert says, nodding toward a man in his forties wearing a red pullover.

"Oh, it's dear," Doris says, "very dear. I don't know how we're affording it. Nice country inns, though, and good pubs, like this one here. They've done it up right for us. Good inns, good pubs. Good thing we're walking it off." She laughs and pokes Albert in the shoulder.

British pub fare has evolved in the time I've been visiting England. Twenty years ago you could get soup and bread or cheddar ploughman's or chili with garlic toast or haddock and chips. Today an array of goodies is on offer: steak and kidney pie, ham and cheese on baguette, lasagna with salad, quiche platter, scampi on basmati rice, curried chicken and nan bread, venison and a baked potato, fettuccine in a cream sauce, entrecotes de boeuf. All cooked up quite competently. It's no longer an oxymoron to say, *British cuisine*.

We down a second pint and linger on the grassy square, taking snapshots of the church, then clamber back on to our bicycles. We've got fifty or so kilometres to go before our day is done. Shortly after we've started, Kristen calls out to me: "Why is it that you always seem to be cycling uphill immediately after lunch?" Our heads are thick with beer, guts burgeoning with food. I call back to her, "Why is it that you always intend to stretch before getting back on the bicycle but then forget?"

It's south and east out of Snowshill on a hard-packed road, with a lovely wood on the left and a bit of a heath on the right. Soon the pleasant jaunt out of town becomes a steady ascent into a wood on a ridge. Soon we're thirsty. Beer tastes good when you're drinking it, but like all alcoholic drinks, it dehydrates, and before long we're glugging back the water in our bottles. It's 2:00, the height of the day's heat. The sun beats down onto the sheltered track. We're a bit woozy from beer and food, needing to *anaconda*, as our son puts it, rest and digest. But instead we're pounding along dirt tracks that dip and rise, climbing and then descending, climbing and then descending.

Our route goes past Stanway, then Hailes. There's a square of grass at the centre of these villages: benches, wildflowers, and a giant yew spreading shade. Trim gardens front most residences. Purple, pink, and rose blooms trail from the golden stone fence work. Stunning quiet. You sit on the grass to do some stretching and what you hear is the birds in the trees and the pit-pat of water dripping somewhere. In the distance a door clicks shut; a small voice echoes briefly: "... and remember to put out the dog." Otherwise the only sound is your own breathing. You lie back on the grass and study the formation of grey clouds overhead: is this "early mist, then mainly fine"? In one way, you have to admit, it's heaven.

You pedal the rolling and winding tracks and lanes hour after hour, smelling hay and marshes, and the ripe pungency of cow dung; gape at panoramas of hedgerows and forests and sunny meadows. You note the winking river in the valley, and on the hills the fluffy white sheep. You negotiate an occasional roundabout and bump along the quiet High Street to get to an attractive inn. One pint of bitter between the two of you, a packet of crisps. The friendly man behind the bar with the starched white shirt and winking spectacles leans toward you and says, "Canadians, is it? We thought you were American. Don't much like the Yanks."

Then it's past a ruin of a castle and a pause for the view of the manor house, now a National Trust site. It's scoot along the track behind the hospital and gape at the wrought iron gate of the boarding school, boys wearing red and yellow and blue and green jerseys running on the fields, their voices high and excited. It's rattle over a wooden bridge, gawk at an ancient aqueduct, dip into a shallow ford, cool water splashing your feet, climb a long hill, puffing, then slow the pace for the farmer in a Land Rover herding his cows from one pasture to another across the dirt track. You wave, he waves back.

At the bottom of a short hill there's a stream that requires jumping, and then a climb begins. You stand up on the pedals for a minute or more. Time to sweat off the beer. The climb is steep. Past a barn. Trees overarch the route, mercifully blocking out the sun for short stretches. There's a celebrated prehistoric burial site here, Belas Knap, but at the height of 1000 feet, with more to go, you keep on pedalling. You're sweating, and not only from the heat. Three towering electrical masts hover in the view directly in front of you. Flocks of birds whirl up from the fields, which are dotted with red-flowering plants, like poppies. A stone wall, in the distance a golf clubhouse, a cluster of red-brick buildings and you top the summit, sweating, heart hammering, hands trembling. The highest point in the Cotswolds. Stunning views of the rolling countryside and then an unnerving escarpment below, Iron Age campsites. You've read about the site of a Roman villa nearby, complete with intact mosaic floor, and you make a note to check that out. But it's 4:10 and supper in Stratford is on the menu for the evening.

Stratford: the place where the street (*straet*) fords the river (*afon*).

A handful of charming pubs in Stratford serve wholesome meals in the evening. But the number of trendy places, complete with winking and blinking video machines, "Italian" menus, ales from the industrial giants, and piped-in pop music is depressingly high. Always crowded with under-thirties on the make, these places are more likely to have Bud on tap than genuine ale. They are noisy, smoky, and crowded. We poke our noses into one, then another. TVs riveted to metal stanchions in one corner blare the sounds of Hollywood B movies over the roar of conversation. No one is watching. The food comes out of aluminum foil packages and goes directly into a microwave oven: Swanson's TV dinners on a commercial scale.

We spot a modest-looking trattoria close to our hotel, the King's Arms, and plump for that. But first a pint or two at the bar.

DEAD MAN ON A BIKE:

UP MOUNT LEMMON

Once you become fearless, life becomes limitless.
~ Unknown

Grinding up Mount Lemmon, Tucson, Arizona. A sunny Saturday morning.

Beside him an old hockey pal, Bill, come over from California to give the famous mountain a try. Two old farts putting themselves to the test.

At the bottom it's sunny and warm, but as they climb to five and then maybe seven thousand feet, it gets chilly, so they've brought windbreakers for the descent.

Clicking through the gears in the first kilometre, Dead Man on a Bike asks, "What cadence you hoping to set?"

"Eighty," Bill replies, "but I don't think I'll manage."

Up and up. With a cheery *mornin'*, a young woman goes by them, bent low, aero bars, a time trial bike, that hollow *burrr* of disc wheels. What the fuck! Climbing a mountain on a time trial bike? Who is this, the famous American pro? Beside him Bill is labouring. Check the heart monitor: 146. They're not working hard aerobically but they're grinding it out. He's already felt his sacroiliac give a sharp twinge.

A slug of water. He had coffee before leaving but the taste is gone.

Starbucks in two hours. Where is Kristen at this hour? Back in "Winterpeg", working, maybe on her bike, even though it's just +5C there with an ungodly prairie wind. Wind is the prairie version of mountain. Climbing the wind, climbing Mount Manitoba. Who was the wag who remarked: *the wind is never with you—it's either against you or you're having a good day?* If Kristen were here ...

Getting a woody on a bike is not a good idea.

This is how you think on a bike. Fast flashes of mentation. Brilliant observations you think you've never had before, no one has ever had before. I should write these down. Later you recall one and think, What the fuck?

Five kilometres. He asks Bill: "How you doing?"

"Got a cramp," Bill says, "something I ate last night." But he keeps turning the pedals. He's not getting off the bike, he's not giving up. A guy coming down the mountain whizzes by on the left; then two young guys go past on the way up; at the end of the next kilometre an older guy on a new S-Works frame. He gears down as he overtakes them—*ka-chunk!* DMB will never understand that— buy an expensive frame and then kit it out with a low-end mech. Would you buy a hybrid Porsche?

Climbing. After about five kilometres the body begins to ask, Why are we doing this? At ten it starts to send messages along the spinal column: Enough already! You say: Shut up, body. To climb you have to turn off the body. Anaesthetize. Pretend it ain't happening. The famous cyclist said: Riding the Tour de France is 3000 kilometres of pointless suffering. Had that right, the bastard.

Ten kilometres. He feels his hips protesting. He's gonna pay for this: sleepless nights, Celebrex, chiropractor. Beside him, Bill is labouring. Another older guy pedals past, puffing hard, rocking on the bike, sweat pouring down his cheeks. It's old farts day on Mount Lemmon. "Maybe we should stop," he says to Bill.

"Yeah, maybe."

Eleven kilometres, 5000 feet of altitude. *Basta*, the Italians say: enough.

In the early '90s the Antelopes give way to lighter mountain bikes: aluminum tubing, rock shocks, index gear shifters on the bars. They're expensive, more than twice the price of the Antelopes, a layout of cash I would not have imagined making in the days of the Peugeot, now hanging for a number of years from a hook in the garage and gathering dust. But swishy: Kristen's green, a Giant, and mine blue and white, a Trek.

We ride them on whatever tracks we can find in the city: along the Red River through the Churchill area from our neighbourhood in Fort Garry to the Forks; over the abandoned railbed in Charleswood, running from Kenaston out to the westernmost reach of the city at the Perimeter Highway—and beyond into Headingley; north from the Forks skirting the river again and into the Kildonans. Weekends we load them onto the car and drive out to Birds Hill Park or the Sandilands or Roseisle, about an hour's drive west of the city, past Carman into rolling hills. One time we venture as far west as Lavenham.

It's a bright sunny day with temperatures in the low twenties Celsius, perfect for off-road riding, the wide gravel road we're on pitching up and down nicely, with challenging short climbs and exhilarating descents, numerous sweeping bends, some of them on downhills: *wheee*. About fifteen kilometres into the ride the texture of the road surface begins to change. Stony grey gravel gives way to reddish hard-packed clay, and at the bottom of a descent the clay turns into mud. We lumber across a narrow bridge. It has apparently rained in the area recently, though the sun is bright overhead, hot, with warm breezes. We begin the climb on somewhat squishy mud; with little warning and approaching halfway up the hill, the bikes begin to slip and slide in the mud. The back wheels start to spin, the front forks are clogging up with thick red clay, we're in danger of taking a header. Halfway up the hill, Kristen can no longer turn her pedals. She de-cleats and jumps off her bike. I am ahead. I hear her choke out: "What the hell!" I dare a quick glance back and see that she's ankle-deep in the thick red mush. Though I continue to pedal, my bike has slowed to a standstill, and before I fall over, I have to concede to the conditions and jump off, too. In a moment I'm ankle-deep in mud. "Jesus H!"

It is almost impossible to move the bikes, even to push them forward. The wheels are thick with dirt, the forks clogged so the wheels will not spin, our shoes are elephant feet, huge clumps of clay, each seeming to weigh twenty pounds. We hoist the bikes onto our shoulders and make for the verge of the road, which is composed of rough gravel, long scratchy grasses, and low spiky shrubs. By now the bugs have moved in: bluebottles, wasps, mosquitoes, the dreaded and horrid horsefly, which takes a chunk of skin when it bites. With sticks scrounged from the verge we set to work scraping gobs of clay off the wheels and out of the forks, and cleaning our shoes, all the while batting at the flies and cursing. We are hot, sweaty, and pissed off.

Swearing seems a waste of energy. Tempting as it is, we do not hurl the bikes into the woods.

From the bridge below us we hear an approaching car. It begins the climb up the muddy hill, slip-sliding and throwing mud from its wheels. It's an old red and white Chevrolet, a heavy vehicle with a powerful engine and a decade and more of rust spots along its wheel wells. As it approaches us it's losing speed fast and the driver guns the engine to keep it moving, causing the car to fishtail from side to side and give us a boom-boom bath. Though he has both hands tight to the wheel, the driver gives us a helpless look—what the hell can I do?—and we forgive him the clots of mud that splatter onto our shirts and cheeks, and onto our lips. Spit. Tastes like boom-boom, too. Wipe.

We stagger to the bottom of the hill with the bikes on our shoulders, drop them unceremoniously on the gravel surface, and drink some water while swatting bugs; then we set off back down the road. For five or ten kilometres clots of mud fly off our tires, some sticking to our legs, others whizzing past our faces.

As the track underneath becomes solid gravel again, the occasional stone is thrown up and pings against the underside of the machines. We look across at each other and grunt; then we laugh; whose idea was this? Then to cap off the day's ride, we have a puncture.

DEAD MAN ON A BIKE:

TUCSON THRENODY I

After you die you will be where you were before you were born.
~ Arthur Schopenhauer

At the bottom of a descent, just to the side of the bike lane, a dead rabbit.

DMB sighs.

Yesterday two birds: one dun sparrow, one yellow warbler.

Too bad, little fellas.

A serious case of projection, he thinks, a serious case of anthropomorphism. But what does that mean? A fancy word to dismiss real and painful connections with the animals around us.

He's the Dead Man on a Bike. Diagnosed with a rare cancer in 1994. Given "two to five years" by the first oncologist he saw. Fuck that. Got another oncologist. "You're healthier than me," that one said, "but you've got a terminal cancer. We can't do much about it except try to hold it off." Live with it, was the message.

On the phone, his old pal, Reg, a physician, tells him: "Think of it as a condition. Like diabetes, or Crohn's." Live with it, he's saying. Before hanging up, Reg adds, "Be glad you don't have diabetes."

Terminal cancer: he'll ride into the wind for the rest of his life, now.

Here's a long, gentle descent and he lets the bike go, lets his legs go. This is the fun part of cycling, the reckless half madness of barely controlled speed. As a kid he played hockey and enjoyed the thrill of scoring goals, the camaraderie of teammates and so on. But what he really liked was skating alone on a sheet of ice early in the morning, sprinting between blue lines, cutting figure eights through centre, skating laps backwards. He used to get up early and go out on the rink alone, and now he loves being out on the road alone, the swish of tires, birds calling in the trees, breeze on cheeks, roar of wind in the ears. The loneliness of the long-distance cyclist.

Maybe he's a weirdo. Maybe all cyclists are weirdos.

He's cruising through a long curve and standing without being aware of it.

Somehow he's been riding and thinking, both at the same time, though neither is very clear. When you're riding you have this weird split focus, watching the road for cracks in the tarmac, noting a sharp curve ahead, road furniture, everything is sliding by and you recall little of it, yet at the same time any one thing takes over your mind completely: the lyrics of a song, the look in a girl's eye, what you should have said to your asshole brother.

From the other side of a tall wooden fence comes a woman's voice saying: "flowers." And then a man's voice: "just as I thought … telephone."

Velocity: 42; cadence: 83; heartbeat: 122; distance: 33. Road cycling is all about numbers. What isn't?

Up ahead there's an old geezer in a red cloth cap at the side of the road with a dog on a leash; the geezer decides to cross at shuffle pace. DMB doesn't know whether to swerve in front of him or behind, the old fellow may do anything now, lurch, go back, turn into stone in the middle of the tarmac. The problem is the dog is on a retractable leash and may dash forward, entangling DMB's front wheel in dog and leash. Stupid old bugger. He swerves sharply left, swooshing past the dog; the geezer starts and cries out, "Ah!"

Invisible, he reminds himself, ride like you're invisible; live like you're invisible.

The new aluminum frames are good mountain bikes, light, manoeuvrable, easy to stand on and "hammer," equipped with lots of gears for rapid shifting and altering speeds on ascents and descents. They make a trip to England, and take us along the South Downs Way, Devon, Dorset, Sussex, and across the Salisbury plain: more picturesque villages, delightful pubs, winding lanes and byways, cathedrals—and Stonehenge, "one of the greatest henges in the world." Brambles, lacerations, punctures, a particularly nasty fall along the side of a road where a drainage well is hidden to the eye by matted grasses—straight flip past the handlebars, ass over tea kettle and flat on the back in seconds—thank Dawkins no cars immediately to the rear.

One day a cycling pal tells me about a mate of his, who is a representative for bicycle manufacturers, a man who receives a free mountain bike every year from one of the manufacturers as a bonus. He is selling last year's bike at a good price.

It's a flashy red K2/Proflex 4000 (the two companies are in the process of merging), a bike with a relatively light frame, a rear shock on the down tube and state-of-the-art "Noleen" front shocks. It is a great ride, and at less than half the retail price, a terrific bargain, though "mum's the word," the bike rep points out, as he pockets my eighteen hundred dollars; he isn't supposed to resell his bonuses. It is bright and beautiful and it handles gravel dumpings, mud ruts and rocky descents over boulders the size of small loaves with equal ease. The tires whizz on downhills and the mech clicks through the gears on ascents with wonderful precision. The shocks cushion the worst of the rugged going and make the ride smoothish, if not exactly comfy.

There are crashes. You don't ride a mountain bike without slipping out on a sandy corner or misjudging rock piles for a mouthful of dirt. But mostly this is a bike that is ridden as a cross-bike, out past the city limits on gravel and mud tracks, across farmers' fields, along riverbanks, country riding where the landscape gives way to boreal forest and the sky overhead is bright blue and the only sounds are the whizzing of spokes, the chattering of birds in bushes, and your own sporadic puffing. You forget the cares of the urban life, its stresses and strains, you shed the snakeskin of the city.

One day I'm on the Trans-Canada Trail running east-west through Charleswood as far as Beaudry Park out on the western edge of the city. Just past the water tower at the town of Headingley, I flat out. It's a hot July day. I flip the bicycle upside down in preparation for repairs. But instead of beginning the repair at once, I sit on the trail and take a long drink from the water bottle. It's hot, I'm sweaty, I'm dry. I'm thinking of Wordsworth: *idyllic and bucolic* flit through my mind. In less than a minute bluebottles buzz around. Where were they before I sat down? Ants crawl on my shoes and up my leg, ticklish. A black beetle with lengthy antennae lands on my arm—bright orange underside, antennae waving in the air. Mosquitoes circle my head, buzzing. Two tiny blue butterflies land on my shoe as one—are they mating? Grasshoppers, more bluebottles, and now the smaller flies, the ones that bite, and a deer fly, then more droning mosquitoes. I have been sitting less than five minutes. Soon these creatures will start to bite. They will drive me away. *All right,* I sigh, standing, abandoning Wordsworth and his recollections in tranquillity. *You win.*

One day I'm cycling down a gravel road just past the junction of the Perimeter Highway and Wilkes Boulevard. A highway crew is working on the verge of the road, digging a hole, maybe repairing the shoulder. These items are in my line of sight: a few stunted bushes along the ditch; in the distance a hydro-electric tower, so far distant the power lines cannot be discerned; gulls swooping near the overpass. Otherwise, blue sky and the big prairie sun. The highway guys are wearing orange reflecting vests and bright canary hard hats. They are the tallest thing for miles around. What is going to fall on their heads?

One day I'm riding along a dirt road west of Highway 75, near St. Adolphe, heading west. It is two o'clock on a summer afternoon. One cloud in the sky overhead. When I pass under it, a light rain falls. After no more than a hundred metres, the rain stops. My shirt is soaked through, but not unpleasantly on a hot afternoon. The rest of the ride is uneventful. The next day I am at exactly the same place at the same time: one purplish cloud overhead: it drops rain on me. What the hell? Two weeks later I have forgotten these odd conjunctions and am riding the same road at the same time of day, two o'clock, I'm lost in thought, musing about the CT scan I'm scheduled to go in for in a couple of days: I've been experiencing gut pains, my family physician thinks a few tests are in order. A dark cloud overhead drops rain on me for no more than two minutes, soaking my shirt through. I hop off the bike and stand on the road, arms akimbo, head tilted up at the otherwise blue sky. "All right," I yell, "you've got my attention. What is it you want to tell me?"

One day I'm on the gravel road just past the town of Heading-ley on the south side of the Assiniboine River, heading toward Beaudry Park. The water tower of the Headingley Jail heaves into view and I think, *Jonny*. Always when that water tower comes into view I think *Jonny*. He was a school pal of my son, Andrew, Jonny, who was struggling in school years ago when they were twelve or so, always rolling the ball uphill, Jonny, getting into fights in the schoolyard, sassing back teachers, living life the hard way.

Most of the time when you're on a bike your mind is either totally engaged with the road—cracks in the surface, upcoming signs, traffic—or in a kind of reverie of blankness, *tum-dee-dum*. But there's also this: years ago when I first spotted the water tower at the Jail, I was thinking about Jonny, and every time since then, no matter what else is going on in my life, when I spot that landmark I think: *Jonny*. I may not have thought of him for a year or more; I don't know what's happened to him. Jonny could be a drug addict, he could be in law school. But I see that water tower and whatever I happen to be thinking is gone; I think Jonny, and for a few minutes my mind spins back to those days long past when Andrew and his pals were in junior high and played on the local soccer team, the "Carrots," coached by Kristen: so much joy in the game, so much promise in their young bodies. *Jonny*. The human mind. Twenty thousand years of evolution and we still don't know why we think what we think when we think it.

One day I'm riding along a gravel road, south of the Brady Landfill site, going east to west. It's a hot July day. My legs feel strong; there is little wind. I am in a dreamy zone, half trance, half sexual fantasy. Bike fog. I've come ten kilometres. After another three I decide to take a road to my right and head north, intersecting, I presume, with Wilkes. I have never been down this road. I bounce along the rough gravel. One kilometre, two. Blackbirds call from the ditches, a hawk swoops overhead. Occasionally a 4x4 speeds past, stirring up dust. My water is running low, but I am dreaming, lost in reverie, not unusual for cyclists, not unusual for me:

I've taken up meditation since my cancer diagnosis and I often reach a Zen-like blankness on the bike. Soon I must hit Wilkes. I have travelled almost twenty kilometres. The sun beats on my neck. I am dehydrating. It must be ninety degrees. Up ahead in a bluish shimmer I detect cars on a road, semi-trailers whooshing past. That must be Wilkes. It takes me twenty minutes to get there. It's pavement, not asphalt; it's a divided highway. I don't know where I am. I'm lost. Far in the distance I spot a giant green highway sign, in the direction I think must be east. I ride towards it: semis swoosh past; the sun beats down; my calf muscles are tightening; I'm a bit dizzy from heat and dehydration. When I approach the sign I see I'm on the perimeter, just north of Oak Bluff. Wilkes is many kilometres to the north. I ride kilometre after kilometre. It's 3:00 in the afternoon, hot and dry. When I reach the underpass at Wilkes and the perimeter I find the first shady spot I've seen in almost two hours. I lie on my back in the shade. Heart pounds, head spins, neck burns. Water. I have become lost on the flat prairie! After ten minutes I cycle on, coming after a few kilometres to a golf driving range in Charleswood where I buy a Gatorade with the emergency loonie I carry. The young man behind the counter says, "You don't look so good, dude, you're a little green around the gills." I drink the Gatorade outside in the shade, mop my brow. Push through the remaining ten kilometres home. I've done eighty kilometres in the heat when I intended to do twenty; I suffer a heat exhaustion headache. The next day I buy a compass.

One day I'm on a back road to the east of St. Adolphe, bumping along gravel, sending dust swirling up behind me. Meadowlarks call from the grasses, frogs chitter in the ditches, a dog in a farmyard barks when I pass by. On a telephone sit three crows. They bark out at me as I'm passing: *caw, caw, caw.* I call back at them: *caw, caw, caw.* And laugh. I know the references to crows in classical litera-ture, the way they're dark portents. Two remain on the telephone line but one swoops down and drifts alongside me for a hundred metres, two. It's flapping hard and it flies up onto the telephone line ahead of me. When I pass, it barks out: *ca-raw, ca-raw,* louder than before and seemingly angry. I laugh. I shake my fist in the air. When I'm past I let out a long screech: *cawwww.* This time when the crow swoops off the telephone line it dive-bombs, coming within a couple feet of my head. *Ca-raw, ca-raw.* I duck my head, I pedal on, I keep silent.

One day I go over a nasty crack in the blacktop and the chain jumps in such a way that it strikes the frame of the bike: *ka-chink.* "Ka-chink," I say aloud as I ride on. Fifty metres pass. I find I'm saying in my head, *ka-chink, ka-chink, ka-chink.* It has become an ear-worm, like the line of a song you cannot shake out of your brain: "roller girl, don't worry …" *Ka-chink, ka-chink, ka-chink.* I try to con-centrate on the road, try to think of other things, sing a few bars of a song over and over. One kilometre passes, two. I'm mulling over the supper I'm going to cook in the evening, chicken caccia-tore, and the wine to go with it. The pedals keep turning. I'm in the country, on a hard mud-packed road, crickets in the ditch, crows on the wing, the rumble of a tractor in the distance. I stand up to take another position, to relieve the pressure on the tailbone. When I sit back down I'm running my tongue over the cavity of these words: *ka-chink, ka-chink, ka-chink.*

One day on the highway that runs through St. Norbert a black pickup goes past me so near that I feel the heat from its exhaust, warm on my hands and face; the frame of the bicycle trembles slightly, a shiver runs up and down my spine. "Close, that was close," I say aloud, "too close. I'm going to die out here."

DEAD MAN ON A BIKE:

WHITE CROSS ON THE ROADSIDE

Everything must be learned, from talking to dying.
~ Gustave Flaubert

Out past St. Adolphe on Highway 200, heading south toward Ste. Agathe, a hot afternoon in early July, just days before going to Edmonton for yet another radioisotope treatment. Hot: 28C, humidex 32. Whatever that means. Sweat on the brow, it appears, sweat on the forearms.

Heart rate: 128; velocity: 27.5. Easy riding.

St. Adolphe, Ste. Agathe, these used to be prosperous little towns: restaurants, auto dealerships, general stores. The churches are still functional—Roman Catholic, exclusively. Everything else: dying.

A tractor belching in a field, crows hopping about at the side of the road.

Here's one of those little white crosses in the verge of the road, plastic flowers at the base, a name painted in black on the white crosspiece. Rest in peace. DMB swallows hard.

Cyclists die; motorists die, hikers die, bikers die. We're not unique, but we're hit often—sometimes, DMB fears, intentionally. Are we ready to die? That is the real question, Hamlet. Not what awaits us after death: Have we learned how to die?

Was it Stendhal who said, "Everything must be learned, from talking to dying?" May have been Proust. Will have to look it up. In any case, there are no tutors to teach us how to die, no old pros who've done the tour time and again and can impart their special knowledge—wisdom. But that is what we're doing willy-nilly: learning to die. Or not. Some folks are just happy to have it happen: good for them—go along in blithe ignorance, then drop off. Or so it seems. But he doesn't believe it. His father often said, "Just let it be fast." And he got his wish: died of a heart attack after taking a pee when he came in for lunch from working on his car. He'd thought it out, he'd moved from Denial to Acceptance in Kübler-Ross's famous taxonomy. In his own way he'd learned to die.

Slug of water. Overhead a hawk riding a wind current, a sweet odour coming off a field of canola.

His father-in-law, near death from cancer, answered his daughter's question, "Is there anything I can get you, Dad?" with: "Fifteen more years, dear." That was the sum of it. More time. It couldn't be bargained for, though. And he knew it, accepted it, and he died well: waited until the family had gathered at his bedside and said goodbye before closing his eyes for the last time. Closed his eyes, let them go.

These are thoughts that are not a cyclist's friend: these are the thoughts that cause you to mist over and not see a stop sign or drift off the tarmac into the tulee bushes and crash. Perilous thoughts sneak up on you when you see one of those little white crosses by the side of the road, black thoughts.

My neighbour across the lane is a cyclist. Once a competitor, Doug is a bicycle enthusiast: he loves to talk about frames, about components, about adjustments that can be made to saddle posts and handlebar stems that increase the comfort of a ride, about tinkerings with shifters and derailleurs to maximize performance. One day he's in the lane when I return from riding the Proflex. "I like that Noleen shock," he says, pointing at it and smiling. I nod in agreement.

He scratches the tip of his nose. "You do road riding?"

I tell him about the Peugeot. It was getting old, I say, just hanging in the garage and rusting; I gave it to my brother-in-law. "I got a bike you might like," he says.

It's a vintage Bianchi racer, one of a half dozen bikes Doug has hanging in his garage, over a generously appointed workbench. Beautiful Celeste paint job with dark blue lettering: *Bianchi*. Campagnolo components, Modello brakes, a tire pump for fixing flats that attaches to the seat tube: it doesn't work, but it looks wonderful. Bright yellow bar tape that accents the dark blue of *Bianchi* on the top tube. "I'm trying to get rid of a few of these," Doug says, waving his arm around the garage, "my wife, you know … Three hundred bucks."

The Bianchi is lighter than the Peugeot but it's made of chromoly steel, and every crack in the tarmac, every bump in the road shivers up my spine. The comfy ride of the front and rear shock-equipped Proflex is behind me. But the components of the Bianchi sing a siren song when you're pedalling, the shifters fluid, the derailleur clicking through the gears. The wheels whizz on downhills, and when I stand to hammer up ascents, the chain and rear cassette are delightfully responsive. This is a fine machine.

I take it on the road in the neighbourhood, making a fifteen-kilometre loop from Jubilee Avenue to Chevrier Boulevard, very nice riding, good blacktop, little traffic, a few little ascents and descents, lots of gentle curves and bends as the road follows the Red River. It's fun, the road bike cruises easily, the narrow tires create little friction with the tarmac, and the bike holds speed, unlike the mountain bike, when I slow for stop signs or cars parked on the roadside; and when I stand to stomp on the pedals, the gears are responsive and the speed jumps up quickly. It's fun. I recall my days as a youth, zipping around my neighbourhood in Atikokan, the thrill is not gone. There's a freedom and excitement to road riding you only get on a mountain bike during hair-raising descents. When I pull into the yard, my heart thumps in my throat, the ride has been exhilarating. I'm pumped.

At the bike shop a few days later we buy Kristen an entry-level road bike, a Giant Peloton, bright canary yellow with black bar tape and a state-of-the-art shifting system on the handlebars that makes the Bianchi's seem very ancient indeed. We ride together on weekends, first west out to Headingley, a twenty-five-kilometre jaunt from our house to Nick's Inn, where we stop for lunch, then south to St. Adolphe, also a twenty-five-kilometre outing, one way. We're not used to riding in highway traffic, the definitive "roadie" experience, but we become accustomed to it fairly quickly: *zoom zoom* on your left elbow; guys in pickups seem to get some sadistic pleasure coming as close as possible; some drivers toot their horns in greeting, but many more blare horns loud and long, *get off the fuckin' road*—you give them the finger, they give it back, that ain't going nowhere.

The fifty-kilometre return journey is not difficult on the legs or taxing in the stamina department, but takes it out of us in an unexpected way. "My ass hurts," Kristen says, standing on the pedals for relief from the hard saddle. "Tour tooshy," I quip. We discuss getting softer saddles but in the end tough it out. "You'll get used to it," Doug tells me. And we do. Though we soon learn the names of creams to apply to the area and to standing on the pedals for short periods for relief. There are sores and soaking in a hot bath. One day Kristen comes home and says, "What's that smell?" I shrug and grin stupidly and try to change the subject. She comes closer. "You smell like a baby," she says, sniffing the air around me, laughing in a sing-song voice: "Hmmm, what could that telltale odour be? Starts with a zee." We both laugh. I've applied Zincofax, which we haven't used since our son, Andrew, was an infant.

DEAD MAN ON A BIKE:
TUCSON PAEAN I

I will get there first, or they will find my body in the road.
~ James Moore, winner of the inaugural Paris-Rouen
(first organized bicycle race)

A lovely warm day in Tucson, 25C, 82F, they say here in old money.

The Old Spanish Trail runs south of the city, a trail the military used in bygone days. Indeed, another such road roughly parallel to it runs nearby, Soldier Trail.

A nice ride: some hills, many undulations, then a long but gentle climb on good tarmac towards Colossal Cave, a tourist attraction at the base of a mountain.

Kristen and DMB have just passed Rincon Corner and are beginning the long climb that goes to Colossal Cave. High above two hawks circle. Hunting, riding the wind currents? Does it feel like swooping down a long descent, a wild rush, half out of control? Little rodents scoot across the road from time to time. Careful, little guys. Geckos sit on the rocks beside the bike lane.

There's time to think here. But first check the gearing. Big ring on the front, sprocket 21 on the rear. May have to gear down where the climb steepens slightly, about a kilometre on.

Suddenly the smell of coffee. There are houses to their left, a huge barn where horses are boarded and ridden. Coffee, one of the original stimulants of riders—along with brandy and then amphetamines. Those guys were riding hard: 3000 kilometres of punishment, up and down mountains in forty-degree heat and rain and high winds. No wonder the great Jacques Anquetil, winner of several Tours, said when someone asked him about drugs: "You can't ride the Tour de France on mineral water" In those early years riders stopped at bars for jolts of strong coffee and slugs of brandy. It was then a short step to liquid versions of caffeine and doses of bennies, and another short step to *Belgian bidons*: mixtures of amphetamines, cocaine, caffeine, cortisone, heroin, testosterone. Then came human growth hormone and EPO.

Drugs. On TV they're always saying, "Just say no." Do the starlets turning forty who want to look like the babes they were at twenty say no? The sluggers who want to hit fifty homers? Everyone's on the gear. What do you call the two-martini lunch? The dudes in rock bands are on cocaine, the matrons at bridge sip Dubonnets with lime. Richard Pryor did so much freebase he lit himself on fire. Every day another preacher from TV checks himself into Betty Ford. Maybe, DMB thinks, he should take HGH for his cancer; maybe try EPO. What the hell.

When you're on a bike, goofy thoughts pop into your head, scoot around in there vole-like for a few moments, pop out again.

A kid goes by on a Trek. Pumping hard, out on a training ride. Americans buy American bikes: Trek, Cannondale, Specialized, Giant. He doesn't see many Colnago or Cervelo, or the bike he rides, Time. His Porsche. The kid is pushing hard. It doesn't matter what bike you ride, not really; what matters is from the hips on down. Still, nice to ride a good machine. He's never going to drive a Porsche, so he may as well ride one.

Near the top of the rise Kristen suddenly says from behind, "You see that?" DMB half turns: "No, what?" She laughs. "You went over a tarantula just there, big as my hand. At least I think it was a tarantula—huge spider, fuzzy legs." He grunts. "Saw my front wheel go over something, thought it was a clump of dirt." She insists: "No, no, it was moving when you hit it, squashed it real good." He doesn't feel the wince he feels at the sight of roadkill. Is that good; is that bad? But, Jesus, a tarantula.

At the top, followed by a flattish section going east, then another long but easy climb to Colossal Cave. A nice ride: heart rate 132, velocity 25. Bright day, sun on the back, good road; could it be any better?

"Sex is better," says old pal Dave, a randy bugger and not much of a cyclist.

"Raising a large family," says friend Sylvia, watching them grow, sharing their joys and pains, being *them* as well as *you*.

"Rack of lamb and a good bottle from the Libournais," says Lyle, himself a trained chef. Cheers, Lyle.

"A cup of Earl Grey tea, imperial cookies, and sitting on the couch watching the latest instalment of *Coronation Street*," says sister Kelly. All right.

"Morrissey concert in San Francisco," says Ken, aficionado of disco, as well as Morrissey, Madonna, Mariah Carey, and Metric.

"Sitting on the tussock of grass near our place on the way to Lockport," says writer friend Patti: watching the dance of sun on the Red River, listening to birds in the bushes, contemplating clouds.

"A walk in the woods," says buddy John, birder: binos around the neck, water bottle in pocket, notebook at the ready.

So many "better"s. *Chacun a son gout.* I'll take the bike.

In December of 1994 I'm told I have a terminal cancer, "slow-moving," my family physician says, but terminal. Maybe, he says, there's really nothing to be alarmed about at this point; it's moving slowly and you've got at least five years, and in five years a lot can change. "My guess is," the doctor says, "you'll die *with* carcinoid cancer but not *from* it."

When we tell my mother, she says, "Oh God, cancer, I'm glad your father is not alive; this would have destroyed him." When we tell Kristen's mother, she says, "No, no," and begins to weep. Her mother died painfully of cancer; one of her brothers-in-law is going through chemotherapy. We find ourselves in the paradoxical position of comforting the people to whom we impart the news.

In the first year or two after, we make significant changes in our life. I stop teaching and rely on income from writing and from investments. We change our diet, we change our drinking habits, we become increasingly aware of what triggers the minor attacks that come on in my gut and lay me low for a day or two, make me miserable; even, sometimes, suicidal. My disease is a gut and liver issue, so what goes into the system, how it combines with whatever else is in there, its progress through the digestive tract are the key concerns. We monitor these things; we learn to stay on top of them; we try to control the disease.

Part of the agenda is exercise. In the early '90s cancer patients are given what has been the standard advice for decades: nothing in excess, don't push yourself. What's suggested is walking, easy jogging, stretching, and yoga. But I've been reading that elite athletes have more elevated immune systems than regular folks and decide that since my cancer is not traumatic, I will take the opposite approach to the standard: I will exercise rigorously, with the object of elevating my immune system: hockey in the winter, cross-country skiing, weights, cycling in the summer. So I'm in the saddle almost every day from April to November. I ride long and I ride hard; I log up thousands of kilometres in the summer. It's part of the new dispensation, the program, the regime. It's me doing something, being proactive.

There's a difference between riding to take a break from headwork and riding as a workout: the first is a bit of recreation on a fine day; the second an athletic effort with an objective: building stamina, increasing power, becoming faster in a sprint. And there's the same kind of gap between riding as a workout and pushing yourself. Pushing yourself, you're trying to make a point: about climbing a mountain or setting a better time between two points; that kind of thing. I find I've entered the realm of pushing;

only my pushing is to make this point: I can do this, I can beat cancer. It's an act of defiance. Yeah, weirdo.

On many of these rides I think briefly of my father, who died suddenly of a massive heart attack a year or so before I was diagnosed. At one time, while in the army, he'd been a somewhat beefy man, but after the stresses of losing his business in his late forties, he became thin and wiry and nervous, highly-strung and of quick temper, puffing his pipe as if he meant to choke down as much smoke as possible, and with it the pains of his recent defeats. He could not be described as a happy man in those years, but he was resolved to pursue happiness, which those of us closest to him found an improbably optimistic attitude, given the cards Fate had dealt him. He made plans, he believed in the future; he rarely spoke with regret and he got on with things. On many Saturday nights he and my mother went dancing at the local Legion Hall.

When he crosses my mind as I pedal through the country-side, I find myself whispering with a heavy sigh, "I miss you, Dad." That's about it, a fleeting nod on a fast-moving bike ride, but that mantra-like phrase is the iceberg tip of a glacial subtext that acknowledges and admires in equal measure his amazing opti-mism. He was *determined* to pursue happiness, a salmon swim-ming upstream, seemingly undaunted by the travails that had befallen him and would have crushed most other men.

Unconsciously, I was chewing over the core meaning of his life, of all life, which comes down to how you manage the cards you've been dealt. Not the cards as such, but the way you pick them up and play out the hand. Pissing and moaning is not part of the equation; it wasn't for my father, and has not been for me. I wouldn't say I'm wildly optimistic; perhaps those close to me would not even describe me as optimistic at all; I operate at a more fundamental level, biological, perhaps, in a zone where optimism does not enter in any more than it does with animals as they go about their daily task of survival, like those salmon swimming upstream.

The long hours in the saddle affect me. My weight begins to drop, from 190 pounds to 180 and then 175. I develop weird tan lines, dark brown from ankle bone to mid-thigh and from wrists to mid-humerus. When I go for massage, my therapist looks at the clear dividing line between the dark brown of my ankle and the total whiteness of my foot: "You're down a quart," he says. My torso, once muscular and broad, shrinks; my biceps become thin. I develop a cyclist's body: muscular but slender thighs, lean calves, slight and lanky upper body. "You're fading away," my writer pal Dennis tells me. "You need to drink more beer." On the bike I feel I'm generating optimum power from my much slighter body; I also feel my butt is paying the price for riding the unforgiving chromoly steel of the Bianchi: *jolt* over every seam in the road, *thump* over every crack in the asphalt. When I'm riding, I'm aware of the texture of the road surface: *Arghh*, a drastic change in the composition of the blacktop is coming just ahead—more gravel and bits of rock, less tar, it's like riding on cobblestones—*brrr* up the spine, kilometre after kilometre.

Solution? I buy a new bike. It's carbon fibre and very light, equipped with a triple chain ring and nine gears on the cassette, twenty-seven gears in all, responsive brakes, comfortable saddle, and pedals that you clip into with the cleats on your shoes. It's extremely manoeuvrable and very expensive. There are cars for sale in *Auto Trader* that cost less. But it rides beautifully. And when Scot at the bike shop equips it with a computer that measures things I've never even heard of—average cadence—I'm in "roadie" heaven. Is it turning into an obsession? Is it keeping me alive? I ride it for two months and can't stop talking about it, convince Kristen to buy a comparable machine. We finish out the season and plan a cycling trip to Brittany.

We're deep in the countryside, some kilometres from the town of Josselin in central Breton (as Bretons call it), a bright and warm morning, heat shimmering off the narrow tarmac as we scoot along beautifully maintained roads in this cycling-mad *départmente* of France. Earlier, when we set off, it was fresh and we were wearing wind vests, but we've taken them off and are feeling the full heat of the day. "We should stop soon," I say as I pull up beside Kristen. "Time for lunch." She nods and keeps turning the pedals.

The landscape of Breton undulates. Slopes, hills, fairly steep climbs, breezy descents. Kristen is having fun. She attacks the smaller hills, jumping up out of her saddle, hammering the pedals, an uphill acceleration in a high gear that produces elevated heart rates, sweat beads on her cheeks, puffing. Then down the other side. My weight holds me back on the ascents but takes me through descents faster. We have fun. Cycling is a sport, like cross-country skiing, that we can do together. We tailor our riding to each other's capabilities; though long stretches pass when there is little communication between us, we're pulling in concert, pointing at sights along the road, sharing observations, stopping occasionally for photos; it's a comfortable way for a couple to be together.

On a bicycle there are lengthy periods of freewheeling along, nothing too strenuous happening, no roundabouts to negotiate, no town with its *Pensez à Nos Enfants* signs, no imminent crises, and your mind wanders. You see the cows, you hear the magpies, you smell the lagoons, but you're taking them in on the periphery. For the most part, you're musing, ideas pop into your mind, snatches of song and so on. It can be an oddly meditative experience. Though also at times this leads to disaster: more than one pro cyclist in a goofy mid-afternoon haze, I suspect, has lost focus and gone over a cliff, or bounced through a ditch, or crashed into an adjacent rider.

In the fields the Jersey cows munch on cornstalks. There's been a heat wave and drought in France the summer of 2003; 3000 dead of heat exhaustion in Paris alone; more than 14,000 in France as a whole. In the days preceding our flight over the Atlantic we saw TV clips of bodies being shuffled out of hospital corridors, of atomic energy plants being shut down, of farmers standing beside truckloads of straw imported from Germany and Poland, the grass to feed cattle had been consumed, and in the drought, had not replenished itself. In Breton in August farmers are feeding their herds the stalks of harvested corn. Cows stand in fields munching enormous mouthfuls of long green and yellow vegetation, the tassels and stalks protruding from their mouths like sticks from the mouths of retriever spaniels. Comical, sad, absurd.

This drought is a random natural event but it wreaks havoc on humans.

The thing of it is, it's irrational, life; it's unpredictable even though we try to make it otherwise. You get into a routine and after a while you begin to think, all right, if A happens then B will follow, it always has, it always will, life has a pattern; you grow to think that's how it was designed, that's how it will always work. But the routine tricks you, you start to believe in design, you convince yourself that life is rational, predictable, dependable, and the thing is, it isn't; day turns into night but that does not mean you can count on one blessed thing happening. Regardless, you rely on its predictability, and you come to believe you're in charge of the game, manager of your own destiny. With routine, we think we can eliminate the truly bad, control the highs and lows. But you're not in control of one solitary thing, you're just the guy in the cartoon who looks up to see an anvil falling on his head; you're just a rabbit caught in the headlights; you're not in charge and suddenly it's all over, there was nothing predictable about it. All along you were fooling yourself, you were dreaming, *I'm going to live forever* because yesterday you got up and the coffee machine was perking as usual, and last week the GST cheque came in the mail as it has for years, and two years ago you said if I set aside this and this maybe one day we can buy the new TV and it worked out, but that was just messing with your own head, a fantasy like love and marriage and Hollywood happiness. Life is not predictable any more than it's forever, it's no more rational than lightning.

In the next town Kristen spots the sign Bar de Huîtres, and we pull the bicycles up outside a modest establishment with four tables. A chalkboard sign reads, UNE DOUZAINE DE HUÎTRES, UN VERRE DE 'ENTRE DEUX MARES' BLANCHE: 10 EUROS. A man appears and smiles at us, the proprietor, we guess, a slender man in his forties with a thin beard, wearing a *matelot* shirt in the stripe of the Breton flag, black and white. We sit and order and in two minutes hear the cracking and shucking of shells. First comes brown bread with butter, then the wine, then two dozen *huîtres*. With a shallot and vinegar condiment, slices of lemon. They're magnificent. One, two, smack of the lips, eight, ten, tastes like more.

Kristen asks the man serving us about the eating of oysters in May, June, July, and August. This is a standard saw we hear back home, received wisdom: never eat oysters in a month not containing an "R"—they're off, they're not good. The man grins. "In the early nineteenth century," he says, "There was a great *enthousiasme* for oysters, so much so that the stocks were becoming depleted, the *huîtres* could not replace themselves. People ate too many. It was a tragedy. There was the fear the oysters would disappear. In fact, they did. But before that happened, Napoleon, who started the code of *no oysters in a month containing an R* decreed this so the oysters could rest for three months in the summer, replenish themselves. It has nothing to do with taste. It was all politics, you see, political economy. As it happened, it didn't quite work. The oysters died out, our native ones, but then they were re-seeded. These are Portuguese, see; in some places they are Japanese. Up north, *hein?*"

Whatever, they're damn fine and we order another dozen.

We look up when we hear English voices out on the street: a group of eight Brits walking past. Brits all over Breton, the two countries, France and England, separated by only twenty miles of sea. Yorkshire voices, Cockneys, South of London drawl. We overhear one say, "Even the cheese smells." The Dutch, the Germans, the Belgiques. Not one American voice squeezing *O* into *A* as in *hackey*, or collapsing double *O* into *U*, as in *ruf*. "This War on Saddam thing," Kristen says. "The Americans are taking the rift with the French seriously." Watching TV, we've seen that the US president and the French are miffed with each other. And since 9/11 Americans are wary of air travel. "Yes," I reply, "they sulk when their feelings are hurt." "So do the French," Kristen whispers. So do the French.

"Those were good," Kristen says, licking her lips after the last oyster has been slurped back. She sips her wine. We look around the Bar de Huîtres. We're the only patrons, though earlier a couple looked in and said they would return in ten minutes. "Those were fabulous," I say, "a real treat." "Good," Kristen continues, "but maybe not as good as the Malpeques from Prince Edward Island. These are fat and juicy but salty, you need the shallot condiment to cut the brackish taste. But PEI's Malpeques are perfectly briny and perfectly dense." We finish our wine. Maybe we'll take a snapshot. "Well," Kristen says as we stand to leave, "not to be unfair. They're no better than the Malpeques." I like that in her, boosting something from back home. We Canadians are so deferential, so ready to believe that whatever is foreign is better. As citizens of a country that was colonized, we've been told this so often we believe it on reflex. But there's no better beef than Alberta's, no more culturally open city than Toronto, no better rye bread anywhere than that to be found in Winnipeg's North End, and so on. Before we made the transatlantic crossing we were reading Anthony Bourdain, New York's self-important, gallivanting chef, who visits Brittany with his brother with the sole purpose of eating *huîtres* ("These were very fine oysters. Maybe even the best"). "He's wrong," Kristen says again, "the New York blowhard, wrong to puff these up the way he does. The Malpeques are as good, there are none better."

An afternoon in the French countryside: burbling streams, vistas of meadows, predatory birds riding thermals, church bells, crickets, cowbells, corn swaying in the breeze, bees buzzing, sun on our arms, the pong of pig shit, rodents darting across the tarmac, ducks floating on ponds, dogs barking, ponies nickering, old fellas in cloth caps playing pétanque, road kill, all that riot in the shrubbery you don't really know about—and don't care to. Urgent sex, then sudden death.

You're in the game and then you're out of it, it's that sudden and that total, and for those left behind that utterly traumatic. Today you're eating a jelly doughnut with black coffee and then … nothing. The line goes dead. You think heart attack, you think cancer, but there are so many ways: a train goes off the rails, you slip and pitch down the basement steps, and that's the end of it, that's your story. The line goes dead. Kristen used to say, grinning, "Not me, I'm gonna live forever," and we laughed but that's what we feel down deep, not me, you and you and you, yes, it's obvious, but not me, I'm in the game forever. First it was a friend with a leaky heart valve, then a relative who put a shotgun in his mouth, Dad bent over the engine of his car, a former student who collapsed from an airborne virus. When we were kids the Sisters used to come to the school and say, *the will of God,* but it does not feel that way, it feels the blow to the gut, it feels I can't breathe, it feels what's the point in going on, it feels all right give up then, but you don't, you put your head down for a moment like with heartburn and then you pull yourself together—it's the kids, it's the work—you take one, two, three deep breaths, it's just something beyond reason, you slowly raise your head and you go on, that's it, nothing fancy about it, no theory, no fine philosophy with hundred-dollar words, you're still in the game, you just go on.

One hundred kilometres in the saddle, a dozen oysters in the belly, white wine, an aching shoulder, a stiff back, sores on the butt, sweat on the brow, grit in the teeth and on the palms, tired knees, kinked neck, wind-burned cheeks, Gatorade occluded to the palate, clammy feet, dank hair, glassy smiles. Seven hours in the sun from the time we set out in the cool of morning; once again we've ridden the metric century, climbed, descended, coasted, laboured. We're tired. We anticipate showers and cool drinks and a plentiful evening tuck-in. The bastard with the yellow wristbands once said: *The Tour de France is three thousand kilometres of pointless suffering.* Prolonged and pointless suffering, that's cycling. Hooray for ice packs, back rubs, and Vioxx!

DEAD MAN ON A BIKE:
WINNIPEG PAEAN

The distance is nothing. It is only the first step that is difficult.
~ Marie du Deffand

Winnipeg. It's sunny but chilly, 9C with a light east wind. Not Tucson, with its warmth and pounding sun, definitely not Tucson. Flat, no bike lanes, the roads lumpy and bumpy. The roads of Winnipeg are crap: cracks, jagged rough patches slapped on the tarmac, garbage in gutters, accumulations of sand scattered on corners, perfect for skidding out on. Potholes. Drivers who have no respect for cyclists. Horrible but intriguing, too. A certain element of mild danger is what it all adds up to, a challenge not unlike running a gauntlet.

A squirrel sits on the road edge. Haunches down, nose wriggling, tail up. They must be the most common creature on the face of the earth. This one looks across to the other side of the tarmac, and then glances at the bicycle bearing down, mental calculations in a tiny brain. It's early in the year, the squirrel's reflexes are bound to be sketchy. Don't, DMB thinks; don't try it, little fellow.

He's the Dead Man on a Bike. He empathizes with roadside rodents. It's ridiculous, but that's how it is. He swishes past the squirrel, who's holding ground on the verge. Playing it wary. Good thinking, little buddy.

He laughs. He says after he's past, "I salute you, squirrel."

Along King's Crescent the traffic thins. The river is somewhere behind the trim houses he's passing. Under the shade of the trees overarching the road it's quite chilly, he feels the wind swirling around the collar of his light jacket. Definitely not Tucson, definitely not the desert.

Here's a little ascent. Twenty strokes up, the heartbeat jumps as he stands and levers the handlebars. Descending, he lifts his hands off the handlebars and stretches his back. Thatcher Drive, almost in the country. Two women are out jogging on the shoulder of the road, one in pink, one in powder blue, babes with swaying pony-tails and bouncing little tits. They wave as they pass and he waves back. Looking good, babes. We're alive, he says under his breath; go for it, girls.

It's flat here but lovely, the road winding along the Red River, sun shimmering on water, no traffic, just the hum of the bike's wheels on tarmac. DMB sighs. This is what it's all about, the Zen-like trance of riding, thoughts popping in and out of the brain, the body relaxing, the cares of the day dropping off like a snake's old skin. He takes a glug of water. Just give me this, he thinks: the swish of tires on tarmac, birds scudding over the river, sun danc-ing on water. One more day, one more week, one more year. Just give me this.

To be a cyclist you have to be a fatalist. So much can happen out there on two wheels, kept upright only by your shifting body weight: the bike can hit something in the road, throwing you to the tarmac to crack your skull; it can go off the road, over a barrier, propelling you down a cliff and into the trees and rocks below; a motorist can open a car door right in front of you, *smash*; a vehicle can hit you. Death lurks around every bend when you're out there.

Out past Selkirk there's a dip in the road near the "bridge to nowhere" and as I crest it I see an animal writhing in the shoulder. At first it appears to be a groundhog but closer up I see it's a cat, twitching in the final death throes. Hit by a car. This should not happen. I'm not a fan of cats: they kill songbirds, they shit in my herb garden, they pounce on small rodents, voles—shouldn't voles with their wet, black snouts be granted the delights of their elfin lives? So, no, I don't like cats. But this should not happen. Someone's pet will not be coming home tonight. I pedal past, the cat's tabby body inert, my gut in a knot, thinking of the dog we had years ago, Pip, who did not come home one night, my younger sister in tears for days. May the puppy gods guard and keep you, little buddy.

A hundred metres pass, two.

I get off the bike. This is rare for me. I like to ride and ride in one go, start to finish, ride without stopping, ascend without getting off the saddle, descend in exultation, pedal to the point of exhaustion. Riding for me is rarely just exercise, or a jaunt in the country, or part of a training regimen. It's a full-blown immersion, a going down into the self, an exploration of the *in*, as much as an excursion through the out.

It's why I prefer to ride alone a lot of the time.

Did I say that cyclists are weirdos?

The cat writhing to its death has upset me. It's maybe a trivial thing, the death of a cat, but for the cat its importance cannot even be measured. It had one life, that cat, and that life was taken away from it.

I sit on a little hillock, the bicycle lying in the ditch. I'm looking out across a farmer's field in a westerly direction, to the right a marsh with rushes and ducks paddling about. Crickets chirr in the ditch; frogs croak from the marsh. I like this kind of nature. I grew up in the Shield: rugged granite hills, bug-infested muskeg, dense bush—and even denser undergrowth, mosquitoes. Nature where you shoot moose and come out of the woods with lashes from tree branches on your face. Nature as sparring partner, nature you battle to survive. It can be exhilarating, but it can wear you down, too. I prefer softer doses: undulating hills, green grasses, fluffy clouds, openings in the landscape that give onto views; chittering squirrels, chattering birds. Nature sustains me; has sustained me; and will sustain me. I will keep up the struggle for river water dancing in prairie sunlight in my field of vision, or the twittering of red-winged blackbirds in nearby rushes.

Road rage, exultant descents, grins and smiles of fellow cyclists, harrowing crashes, painful climbs, touching deaths, Zen-like moments of peace. I've come to understand something while riding a bicycle—or I've learnt it again after almost forgetting it. It's hard to live with life. Hard to live life. Most of the time we do one of two things: stifle life or rage against it. Suppress feelings through work or other compulsions; or indulge in fury against those feelings. They appear to be two poles on a spectrum, rage and suppression, but they're more two points on a circle, the noon and midnight positions, opposite in one way but mirror images in another. In an effort to live fully, some people just swap between the two, jumping from rage to suppression, then back again. Neither, in any case, allows us to live in life; both are flights from life—through ferocity on one hand and by denial on the other. Neither allows us to feel feelings and make them a part of daily experience, which can be a risky business because it draws us into the realm of madness. How to live, asks one novelist; how to be, asks another. Feel the moment. Sink into it and become part of it.

We're sitting, Kristen and I, with our cycling friends Liisa and Tristan at a B&B in Ellensburg, Washington. After a vigorous day of riding the hills we've been in a hot tub and are relaxing in the white robes provided with the room. Glasses of red wine in hand. Liisa says, "Those are some scars." She nods toward the scabs on my knee and ankle, visible below the hemline of the robe. A few weeks earlier I'd crashed and acquired "gravity tattoos" on shoulder, hip, knee, ankle. I glance down at them: so recent there's a halo of pink tissue between the reddened welts and the healthy skin, like the aureole of a breast.

"You're proud of those," Tristan says. He has bright blue eyes; they appraise me as he awaits a response.

"I'm, no, I'm ..." I don't know what. I think of wounded heroes in literature: Achilles, Prometheus, Chiron. Hemingway's Jake Barnes, who suffers "the wound of which we *do not speak*." Others. Heroes become heroes *because* they're wounded. Literature is about wounding: all of Dickens; all of Dickinson.

We're all wounded. Some at birth: club foot, missing kidney, walleyes. Or abandoned after birth. Or beaten; neglected by parents; bullied at school; polio, meningitis, scoliosis, mono. So many ways to be wounded. As there are so many ways to deal with wounds. To rise above *the wound*. Maybe, yes, we're proud of our wounds; physical scars, anyway, because they're visible reminders of minor triumphs over them. I will not give in; I will not let this get the better of me; I will rise above.

This book is about *the wound*, about how cancer sticks a knife in your side and says, There, do what you can. What are the options? You can fall over dead; whinge out your days; leave the knife to fester; yank it out and splash blood around; pretend the knife is not there; anaesthetize it; use it to wound others; rage. Attempt to ride it away on a bicycle. There are no visible signs of this wound.

Everyone knows they take drugs, the pro riders. They always have; they always will. The sport is just too difficult for that not to be so. The grand tours are made up of twenty stages, each 150–200 kilometres in length, many of them over mountain passes of twenty kilometres in length, one after the other, three or four a day. In one respect, it's equivalent to doing a marathon race twenty times back-to-back. To get through that nearly kills many riders, each of whom is an elite athlete, the crème de la crème of cycling; many riders consider it the feat of their lifetime in the sport to merely *complete* a grand tour: in excess of 3000 kilometres in heat and rain and high winds over roads that are often lumpy and bumpy and riding hard, at an average pace of forty-some kilometres an hour. They "bonk" from not eating and drinking enough; they collapse at the end of the day and have to be helped upstairs to bed; they crash and get back on the bike and continue pedalling, having scraped their skin, twisted wrists and knees, banged their heads on tarmac: because there are no "time outs" in cycling; if you cannot continue, you're out of the race. It's a back-breaking, mind-numbing sport, requiring amazing stamina and total dedication. To succeed at cycling you have to be "hard." And you need help: in the old days it was liquor and caffeine; then amphetamines and cortisone; now deadly combinations of testosterone, steroids, human growth hormone, and EPO.

The bastard with the yellow wristbands took drugs too. In a highly organized regime and on a highly regimented team where he demanded every rider supporting him also take drugs. He did this in an era when every successful rider in the pro ranks took drugs. In that he was no different. Where he was different was in denying it—even when others turned "whistle-blower"; even when the evidence stacked up by responsible journalists in Europe became irrefutable. He not only cheated; he did that thing your mother said was worse than getting caught stealing cookies out of the cookie jar: he lied about what he had done wrong. That was very bad. But worse was this: along the way he started a foundation for cancer sufferers, and then he became poster boy for the cancer community: survivor and brave champion of clean living and purposeful commitment to post-illness goals. He lied to the cancer world and abused his position; the fact that his foundation does good work should not excuse that shameful behaviour. He duped us because we wanted to be duped, we want to believe that cancer can be beaten, that the story has a happy ending, that the hero is virtuous. We should not forget what he did, we should not forgive him for what he did. We should not forgive ourselves.

Risk taker, then. The cyclist is a risk taker. Risk taking is demanded by the ridiculous machine with two wheels that only stays up when it's moving; demanded by the ridiculous activity that calls for its rider to also be its engine. Risk taking. Not of the highest order. We're not shooting up heroin in a dark back alley. Cyclists are not extreme risk takers; we're not prone to jumping off the roofs of our own lives.

The bike ride is not a homogeneous moment, it is not a smooth transit from point A to point B in one fell swoop. It's broken up by stop signs, breakfast at a diner, traffic bottlenecks, the need to pee, stopping to check the map, red lights at intersections, lunch at a bistro, punctures, photos. The bike ride is fragmentary.

Life is fragments. Though we look back on tracts of time in our personal history as long as decades in duration, and divine in retrospect a sequence leading to where we have arrived, seemingly inevitably, there were forks on the way that have mostly been turns in the wheel of fortune, sending us down one road rather than another: ends of relationships, moves from one house/city to another, career changes, arrival of children, incursions of diseases, encouragement from a teacher that leads to the study of biology at university. Life is not a continuous progress from A to B but a jumble of segments that overlap and occasionally require leaps of faith across chasms of uncertainty. The collage, with its teasing assortment, not the railroad track running uninterrupted from sea to sea, is an apt analogy for life.

The nineteenth-century novel encouraged readers to believe in the myth of beginning/middle/end: our hero (ourselves) was born, grew up and matured, prospered despite setbacks, settled into old age and its wisdom. Dickens' *Great Expectations* is the model; *Les Misérables*. Life formed a smooth arc—from birth to death, with intervening years of development and resolution. But life is not like that. Things fall apart: friendships fade or get twisted by misaligned bitterness; diseases intervene; colleagues die; love flags; parents and children grow apart; a better career comes along. Life's components are a hotchpotch, its progress herky-jerky. It does not always lead to personal growth or moral progress.

The writer records life and life history, but the writer can be seduced into constructing the seamless narrative of the nineteenth-century novel, with its uplifting moral growth and positive denouement, and this gives the lie to experience, which is subject to the whims of fortune and is discontinuous, fragmentary, and often resistant to meaning. Perhaps all books should mirror the collage with its fragments and its bemusing disorder. Certainly mine do. They recall T.S. Eliot's eloquent quip: "from these fragments have I shored up my ruin."

The phone in my jersey bleeps and I pick it out and glance at a message from Kristen: *home late, bad day.* She'll need an extra hug.

My mother, when she was expiring at Riverview palliative centre, needed lots of extra hugs. For eighty-seven years she had been among the most independent and resourceful people. But then over a period of a few months she became one of the neediest, and stayed that way for more than four years. She stopped watching TV, reading the newspaper, listening to the radio. She hated sitting in a wheelchair with the other "inmates" in a circle singing or talking. All she wanted was for us, my sisters and me, to visit every day—at least one of us, if not all three. "Stay longer," she begged, "come again soon," "I miss you." What a switch: from resourceful to desperate.

As infants and then toddlers we had been the needy ones. But over the course of fifty years we had switched positions. In bike races, teammates and competitors alike work together, each taking a turn at the front of the group, providing shelter for those behind, before peeling off to take a rest at the back. It makes me think that all of life is like that: one person in a loving couple is the giving one, but then that changes—an illness, dismissal from a job—and the roles are reversed. Is all of life, then, a matter of role reversal: he who was first becomes last; she who was last becomes first?

Getting cancer can be the best thing that happens to you.

It's life's Punch In The Face, no gloves: bone-crushing, sudden, critical. Your nose is broken, your mouth dribbles blood and saliva, your ears ring. You're down for the count. But you'll never be hit like that again. Like most of us crawling across the face of the earth, you fretted about paying off the mortgage, getting the promotion, winning the babe. Making it. Setbacks gave you a knot in the gut, hard as a bowling ball. Sleepless nights, anxiety attacks, reaching for the bottle. The travails of life ripped you. After the PITF, nothing ever hits you like that again. You've been through the bed sweats, the weeping, trembling hands, blank looks when someone posed a question, the rage. The things that life dumps on you now are just things that life dumps on us:

death of a parent, relationship break-up, career setback. Whatever. Each stops you in your tracks, you stagger backwards for a moment, blink, taste bile in your mouth. But you won't go down again. Cancer has hardened you. The PITF is a survival scab.

And it's given you perspective. Instant helicopter shot. All the things you cared about, worried over—the career, flash car, investments—all of that you suddenly see from the height of a thousand feet. The Wellington Crescent address, Prada shoes, Chateau Cheval Blanc: they now appear as the urgent scrabbling of ants. Paltry concerns, unnecessary fret, a giant waste of time and energy. Those things don't matter. One of the great poets once wrote: "getting and spending we lay waste our powers." He was right about that, Wordsworth, but it takes the PITF for most of us to actually see it. To see that the scrambling to get somewhere, to be someone, all these things, don't matter, they're so much dross. Cancer snatches you up by the scruff of your neck from the vortex of your own desires.

Or it can.

Did I say "fatalist"? Fancy term. To be a cyclist involves a certain amount of willed stupidity. One day when you're hurtling down a mountain pass at 70 k.p.h. you'll hit something on the road and splatter yourself all over it. Or a motorist will open a car door just as you come up to it—and *smash*. Or you'll put down your head for a few seconds and find when you look up that the citydiots have placed a metal sign in the bike lane warning of roadwork ahead—*ka-boom*. You know it will happen: sideswipe, puncture on descent, car parked in the road under a "No Stopping" sign just round a sharp bend, into the tulee bushes after a front-wheel wobble. You have to will yourself out there against the knowledge, you have to pretend it's not going to happen.

In the fall of 2004 we arrange a cycling trip with Vancouver friends, Liisa and Tristan, to the Yakima valley in the state of Washington. We've been on a cycling expedition with them before, to the Dordogne region of France. We meet up one evening, settle into a B&B just outside the small city of Yakima, and in the morning begin a ride called the Naches Ramble. It starts on the flat, cutting through industrial sites and a powerhouse, located along the riverbank of the Yakima River. The road winds delightfully for several kilometres to Indian Painted Rocks, petroglyphs located up the hillside, which gives stunning views of the valley and surrounding farmlands. From above, the terrain below looks dusty and dry, with the river running through it.

On the road below we soon pass the bridge that connects the road we're tracing, the South Naches, to the Old Naches Highway, which runs along the north side of the river, parallel to the route we're following. The rock outcroppings are reminiscent of desert scenes in western movies, stones dark as obsidian. On the opposite side runs the Yakima River, pale green in the morning sun, stone-bottomed and bubbling and frothy, a real challenge to canoeists and kayakers. The road winds sharply, staying parallel to the river, with sudden climbs and exhilarating descents. On a flattish stretch, Tristan drops back to join us. "Great guns," he says, smiling.

Orchards stretch out to our left in the arable fields between the road and the river. Apple trees heavy with fruit, large golden yellow apples. We pull over and walk into the orchard, lift up several that have fallen on the ground, bruised and of no use to the farmer. They're huge, but sweet and delicious, crunchy, tasting of honey and cinnamon. Across the road the variety is different, red and even larger, heavy in the hand and sweet on the palate. Our host at the B&B called these honey crisps. They have a thin skin and juice dribbles onto our chins.

When we return to the bicycles, mine has a puncture. "Crikey," I say, snapping the quick release on the front wheel and zipping off the wheel. I hold it up at a sideways angle and say, "La Pannonie, anyone?" We all laugh heartily, remembering our journey through the Dordogne area of France where I had many punctures, once ruining a tire as well as the tube. We replace the tube, laughing and chattering. Same old story. I wipe my hands on a rag and we're off, ascending for a stretch and then passing alongside an open area where there are picnic tables and a gravel parking lot, Eschbach County Park, a sign tells us. The river makes a wide sweeping curve here and above the road on the hills run a number of horizontal streets densely populated with ranch-style bungalows clinging to the steep hillside. Barking dogs.

Noon approaches. The sun has moved directly overhead and we're sweltering in the heat. "Hot and dry," Liisa says, "I've never felt anything like it." When pickup trucks go by, they stir the dust on the sides of the road. We pause to drink water and wipe our brows. Overhead hawks circle.

Kristen says, "That's some dry. Make sure you keep at the water." We gaze out across the flat farmlands. Orchards, in some places fields of hay where cattle gather round water troughs or shelter under stands of trees. Flies buzz about our heads. The sky is totally blue. It's hot and it's going to be hotter. Sweet and cloying odours emanate from the fertile orchards. The wind sweeps down from the north, ruffling our hair and stirring the autumn leaves in the ditches.

We start to mount up and discover Tristan's rear tire is flat. He's riding an old steel Bianchi that he's been nursing through decades of strenuous trips here and there, and the rear wheel is difficult to remove and even trickier to reposition once the puncture has been repaired. We grunt and sweat. The pannier attached on the rear rack slows our efforts.

"I keep telling him to buy a new bike," Liisa says. She's riding a new hybrid, aluminum frame, bright colours on the down and cross tubes.

"I know," Tristan says, laughing, "I know, I know. I'm just too cheap."

He derives a certain pleasure from bashing along on his old warhorse, even, I suspect, from the travails of maintaining and constantly repairing it. A good part of cycling is the machine you ride, and you grow attached to it, understand its quirks, forgive it its little foibles: a rear wheel that wobbles slightly, a chain ring that squeaks on steep ascents. It can be difficult to part with a machine that has carried you over thousands of enjoyable kilometres. Maybe it takes you back to the time you cycled in Italy with a former lover; maybe your father, rest his soul, bought it for you as a birthday gift many years ago.

Just after noon we cross the busy Highway 12 that has replaced the two rambling roads that run along the river into the town of Naches, pronounced "Naw-cheese" by the locals. It's a sprawling country place, wide streets, ranch-style store fronts, pickup trucks, a water tower, old men wearing soiled baseball caps sitting on wooden chairs under faded awnings, smoking and chewing the fat. We pull up at a modest restaurant, diner really, that has tables outside on the wide sidewalk. "Reminds me of Texas," Tristan says, hooking his thumbs into his shorts and swaggering about in front of the saloon-style doors.

"Pardner," I say quietly, aware that we may be overheard by the locals.

"Look at the flags," Liisa says.

Up and down the street every business establishment flies a Stars and Stripes, some the size of frigate sheeting. We're not used to this in Canada. In Sunnyside, where we stayed a few days, our B&B hostess wore an apron in the design of the US flag. She

and her husband were retired cops, she told us. "We don't understand those people up north," she said, meaning Seattle, "with
their goofy ideas and soft attitudes. We vote one way down here,
they vote different up there." She didn't explain, but the Repub-
lican posters on the walls in the foyer were a good clue. Tristan
and Liisa did not mention they were from Vancouver, a city more
left in its leanings than any in the USA; Kristen and I that we were
from a province that has elected a socialist government twenty
of the past thirty years and has a gay mayor in office.

Over breakfast at a B&B outside Yakima, our hostess, Karen,
engaged us in breezy chatter on a wide range of subjects. This is
one of the attractions of the B&B, getting to know your hosts,
gleaning a little of the inside dope about their lives, the ethos of
the country you're travelling through. Italians are quick to decry
the laziness of government employees, the *statale*; as they enjoy
their lunch, the French discuss enthusiastically what they're
going to eat for supper; the British chuckle quietly over sex scan-
dals and the doings of the Royals. Karen said, "We don't like the
government to be involved in things; from them we want security
and good roads." We nodded and smiled, the polite Canadians.
Best to keep quiet when politics comes into the discussion.

Inside the restaurant we order delicious-smelling broccoli soup
and potato salad with huge wedges of cucumber and radish. The
woman who serves us asks, "Y'all want sodas with that, or what?"
We have iced tea and a couple of Budweiser beer. We carry our food
on trays outside and sit in the shade of the awning. Two middle-
aged men park their pickup near our table and saunter past us,
cowboy boots, wide-brimmed Stetsons. "Y'all havin' a good day?"
one asks. The other tips his hat and says, "Y'all doing it the energetic way." "Nice country hereabouts," Tristan responds. We're
warm in the shade and stretch our legs and backs like lazy cats.

Two cyclists come round the corner from the opposite

direction we arrived from and zip by on bright road bikes, colour-ful jerseys. They wave and we call out, "*Allez, allez.*" Kristen laughs and says, "Wonder what they made of that?"

Before we can answer, we hear a marching band and in a moment it rounds a corner several blocks away and comes toward us. Baton-twirling majorettes, kettle drums, brass of all kinds; the band is made up of teenagers, possibly a high school group. Enor-mous flags carried by slender boys in pillbox caps: Stars and Stripes, the state flag, others we do not recognize. Maybe the high school itself boasts a flag? The sound is deafening when right close. The kids are having a good time: smiling, laughing, cut-ting up a bit. People come out of the shops and clap and cheer. We join in. Go to it, kids. The band prances past smartly and disap-pears round a corner a few streets farther along, their brassy racket trailing behind for a few minutes.

We've lingered and it's almost two o'clock when we head out north, towards the town of Wenas. After just a kilometre of gen-tle climbing the road turns sharply and begins to ascend steeply. We gear down, then farther down. Sweat breaks out on our brows. "The thing is," Kristen wheezes at my side, "the climbs are short but really steep." This one seems to go straight up, possibly at 12 per cent grade. We're working hard, watching Naches below us dwindle to Toy Town size before we reach the summit. The climb is a 100-metre vertical over less than a kilometre and our hearts pound when we pause for a drink of water.

"Lovely," Liisa says, "I love this open and barren country."

"You're a cowboy at heart," I say. "Cowgirl from Finland."

"Rugged," Tristan says. "Wind blown and stagy as a B movie. I expect John Wayne to come cantering up at any moment."

I say, "Better believe it, Pilgrim."

Liisa adds: "I've never seen terrain like this."

Kristen drawls, imitating Tristan's earlier speech, "Nice

country here-bouts." She points into the distance: peak upon peak of brown, rounded mountains. She snaps a photo.

The road winds through farm country, cattle ranches and grain fields along Wenas Creek. The town is tiny but has a charming café and several stores. We circle around and then do the return descent, the breeze cool on our faces. At the bottom Kristen and I look back. Tristan has pulled over to the side of the road. He has a puncture. Back tire, of course. While we do the repair, Kristen examines his tire. Stuck to its outside is a hard kernel, which, when she removes it, reveals two tiny prongs that are sharp as metal staples and look like the pincers of certain beetles, hooked and spiky as the teeth of fish. While we examine it, a cyclist on a mountain bike pulls up.

"Aha," he says, "goatsheads, they're all over the roadside here. Damn nuisance. Even if you're not riding skinny tires, you can't pull your bike off the road."

"That's our third puncture today," Liisa says.

"I hear you. They're a damn nuisance."

"Every time we stop," Kristen adds, "we get a flat."

Liisa says, "What can you do about it?"

"The bike shops have these extra thick tubes that come with a gel inside. So when they're pierced, they close up around the puncture. They make a seal."

"Or don't go off the road," Kristen says. "Stay on the tarmac."

"They're in the grass. Blow off some of these fruit trees or something."

"Sharp little buggers," Tristan says. "We're using up our spare tubes."

When we resume our journey, the road undulates through farmlands—orchards below, between the road and the river; pastures and meadows above. Lovely views of winding, sparkling waters, green slopes, cattle. In the distance the rounded brown

---

hills and much farther distant the snow-capped crest of a mountain. "Mount Rainier," Tristan tells us.

Terrific riding, though the tarmac varies from smooth and flat to crumbly and potholed. The orchards are fertile. Pungent odours of the harvest waft by on the breezes. When we glance upward toward the slopes on our left, we see the fields have been irrigated extensively with trenches and metal piping. Farther south, around Sunnyside, where every second field is grape vines, the land is irrigated by giant sprinklers that cast spray up to 200 metres in every direction—refreshing if you're on a bicycle under the blazing sun. The Yakima valley, once renowned for its many fruits, is now earning a serious reputation for solid red wines: cabernets, shirazes, merlots. We've sampled a number and they compare favourably to the Aussie products. And here in the valley itself, they're available for as little as $6 per bottle.

Through the village of Selah and then across the bridge that connects the Old Stage Road to the South Naches, and it's back on the winding passage that leads to our B&B. There's a moment outside when we share high-fives and talk briefly about the beauty of the ride: the undulant terrain, the emptiness of the roads, the smells and sounds of the Yakima Valley. One of the best rides we've done together, we agree. Maybe before our riding begins tomorrow, we think, we'll visit a local bicycle shop and buy those gel tubes.

For now, we'll relish the dinner we've planned at Gasparetti's, an Italian restaurant in Yakima, where, our hosts tell us, they do a terrific osso bucco and mouth-watering ravioli. The food sounds as if it would go well with one of the reds we've tasted at the wineries in the Sunnyside area.

DEAD MAN ON A BIKE:

A SMALL PASSAGE

We cannot learn without pain.
~ Aristotle

They're breezing along a county road in rural Wisconsin, a hundred or so kilometres east of St. Paul, Minnesota. The road is in a valley, county road X. In this part of the state, east of the Mississippi, several counties that form the border between Wisconsin and Minnesota, ridges run north-south every few kilometres, a landscape that from above must resemble corrugated cardboard. Some five or six kilometres back they came down a descent, off a lovely ridge ride, a whooshing, exhilarating downhill of some four kilometres, with many sharp bends, gravel and sand crunching beneath the tires, fun but dangerous. Wheee!

The riding on the flat is pleasant—and never quite flat. Always there's a little undulation ahead, a gentle descent just behind. This is farming country, the heart of America: fields of corn and soy beans, Jersey cows grazing pastures, hay bales stacked in fields. A silent landscape: only the sound of crickets and tinkling cowbells, the whirr of their bicycle tires; in a nearby field, a tractor making hay bales, chuffing diesel into the air.

Hawks circle overhead. One suddenly plummets into the field ahead of them, lands, hops about. "The tractor must stir up the mice," Kristen says, "while cutting the hay."

When they approach, the hawk flaps off. DMB tries to get a photo but what comes out is a black smudge against blue sky.

The road is smooth tarmac, very few cracks, no frost boils or potholes. In the USA they take care of their roads. This one goes up and down, terrific undulations for bike riding, long sweeping curves, almost no vehicle traffic. "Wonderful ride," DMB says between sips of water.

"Glorious," Kristen says. "Not a cloud in the sky."

"Sounds like a metaphor," he says, laughing.

A tractor approaches, pulling a piece of farm equipment—a mower? The farmer lifts one finger off the steering wheel in greeting. They wave back. There are silos in the distance and giant slurry tanks, and when they descend into a bottom, the pong of cow dung momentarily takes his breath away. "Wouldn't want one of those babies springing a leak," he says, of the slurry tanks. They both laugh. At a junction they join County U, a slightly busier road.

They pass a milk-processing plant. It's a pretty big operation; twenty or thirty employee vehicles parked out front, semi-trailers with bright steel tanks attached, idling motors in a parking lot. The tankers prowl up and down this route, bringing raw milk from nearby farms and carting processed product away.

Crows on the side of the road. They must be the most common creature on the face of the earth. When they pass the next farmyard, a big woolly black dog starts up from behind a bush, whoofing loudly as it charges across the open space toward them. They're moving too fast for it to catch them, but DMB's heart rate accelerates. They catch you by surprise, these unleashed farm dogs, give you a bit of a fright.

When he and Kristen are several hundred metres clear of the dog, he says, "Don't think he really meant it."

"No. It's the little yappers I can't stand."

"Punters."

"Yeah. Need to be punted back into their yards."

They chuckle. Saying these things is a kind of exorcism; it's unlikely either of them would kick a dog.

The town they're staying at is only a handful of kilometres distant. End of the day's riding. A good day. There's a bungalow beside the road up ahead, mowed lawn, a flagpole with the Stars and Stripes drifting in the breeze. As they come up to it, a black kitten comes staggering from the shallow ditch toward the road. It teeters weirdly, one step, then a second; on the third step it lurches awkwardly sideways, and then it falls over into the grass. Inert.

"Did you see that?"

Kristen says, "It just fell over."

"I think it died. Just like that. Keeled over."

"Should we go back?"

They check behind them. Three milk tankers are just to their rear; they cannot easily double back. The tankers swoosh by; they grip the handlebars tight, feel the road shake, Dopplered by the trucks' drafts. A kilometre passes; another quick shoulder check. They don't turn back.

"That was really weird," Kristen says. "It just keeled over."

"Defunct. Geez. One of the oddest things I've ever seen."

They sip water in silence.

"A small passage."

"A little death."

Yes, the first thing you think upon being diagnosed with cancer is, Why me? It seems so unfair, as the deaths of children are unfair, as the deaths of friends at an early age seem unfair. At any age. "Everybody gets cheated," my writer pal Dennis says, and he's right. So, you're going along, enjoying life, making plans, building a life with someone, having children, perhaps, generally feeling good, except for that nagging headache you get every now and then just behind the ear, or whatever. The headache returns; it occurs more often; you visit your family doctor, who sends you for a CT scan. All seems in control, just routine, eliminate the unlikely. But the bad thing isn't eliminated. There's a tumour and it's on the move and it may be fatal, so you have to go in for this test and that procedure, and not next week or next month, but tomorrow, and it's not benign; you haven't been sleeping that well as it is, and now your nights are wholly restless and filled with nightmares, you wake crying out, and you develop constipation, or diarrhea, and black marks develop under your eyes, your increasingly puffy cheeks itch in an inexplicable way, and, yes, it's malignant. Only a month has passed since you went in to see your physician and you may have only months left. Jesus, the job, the career, the kids, the renovations, the will. Why me?

For a week or two, maybe a month, this is the constant refrain. It's totally and absolutely understandable—and an entire waste of time. Why me? is something you have to get past. I'm heartbroken every time I hear of someone who is diagnosed and does not make it past six months. For me, that's a magical date. If you can get out that far, past the six-month point of hearing *you have cancer,* there's a chance you will develop some perspective, catch a mental breath, so to speak, regroup, put life in perspective. Rise above the horrid question: Why me?

It comes down to luck. If you're lucky enough to get a cancer that does not do you in immediately, there's a chance. Lucky enough, did I say? It does not sound like luck to get any type of cancer, but it can be.

Why me? can be followed by: what can I do? And that's the first step to getting a handle on life again.

Following my diagnosis, I read a lot. Books, pamphlets with discussions specific to my cancer, articles in learned journals, newspaper clips, whatever I could lay my hands on. In one of those books, an oncological surgeon, Bernie Segal, makes the following observation, which struck me at the time and has stayed with me since: Segal says that his patients fall into three categories: those who take their diagnosis as a signal (maybe he says "excuse") to die; those who say to their physicians, I'm not having anything to do with this (it's up to you to fix me); and those who say, What can I do? In his experience, this last group contains the greatest number of survivors.

Where do we go from here? Start from the bottom, back to basics.

If you like hiking or walking, put on your shoes, drive to that quiet stretch along the river where you enjoy spending an afternoon: fluffy clouds overhead, the singing of blackbirds in the rushes, water sparkling in the sunlight. Walk until the worst of that knot in your gut starts to loosen. Enter into the zone that for lack of a better term can be called *peace of mind*. The Zen of motion and *not-thought*, or not the thinking that is primarily anxiety and fear and despair, the zone where you feel your oneness with the natural world and the blessing that life is, the Zen of moving down into yourself. There's a bottom. And at the bottom, it's all up from there.

If you have a bicycle, get on the bike. Go to that spot where the traffic thins and reflection thickens and releases you into what was once called "the peace that passes all understanding." The poet Keats, aware that he would die, as had his siblings, from tuberculosis, begins one of his most moving poems this way: "When I have fears that I may cease to be ..." After considering such fears and frets for a dozen lines, he concludes the poem by saying: "... then on the shore of the wide world I stand alone, and think Till Love and Fame to nothingness do sink." He nailed it.

Of course, you can go crazy too: climb Kilimanjaro; sail around the world; blow your RSP on a spending spree; travel the world to see what there is to see; try parasailing and bungee-jumping and skydiving; dine at the finest restaurants and drink only the celebrated vintages. There's a "wild and crazy" guy inside us all, and this may be the time to let him take the bit in his teeth.

Most of us do not go that route. A few of us commit suicide.

There are things to be done, things that make for a better life than wallowing in "Why me?" They come from these questions: What can I do, where do we go from here, how do we proceed? They take courage, and there's no guarantee they'll work, and they do not cure the condition. But they can make meaningful life possible. For some they are the door to meaningful life; it's not unusual to hear cancer patients say, *cancer was the best thing that ever happened to me.*

Here endeth the sermon.

DEAD MAN ON A BIKE:

DE MORTS PETITS

Death is not an artist.
~ Jules Renard

November 12, the day after what they call Veterans Day in the USA, back home called Remembrance Day. Poppies, twenty-one-gun salutes, the mother of a fallen soldier laying a wreath at the cenotaph in Memorial Park. We try not to forget their sacrifice. My father, a bombardier in the anti-aircraft; he did not see action; his unit was set to ship out from Vancouver Island to the Japanese islands when war in the Pacific ended. An uncle I did not know cut down on the beaches of Normandy. When my mother, pregnant, opened the telegram that confirmed "missing in action," she miscarried. A little death.

DMB is out on the road in Tucson. Nine o'clock in the morning. A slight breeze to the rear, a bright sun overhead. 56F (14C), chilly, but by mid-afternoon going to 75F (22C). The roads are busy: commuters hustling to jobs, school buses picking up children, light trucks heading to work sites. At certain times of day the cars on the left elbow of cyclists seem closer than at other times; maybe it's the constant whirr of rubber on asphalt; maybe they do actually crowd the bike lanes more. Whatever, it's an unnerving time to be out on the blacktop. School buses especially seem to drift dangerously close.

DMB makes the turn off North Sabino and is heading west on Sunrise. The road climbs gently here, so gently it's almost not noticeable. Here's a dead bird in the shoulder, mashed already by the pounding of numerous car tires, feathers sticking up every which way. Black? Difficult to tell as you pedal past. Could be a crow, a larger bird, in any case. They're hit occasionally. DMB sighs.

The turn north at Kolb Road begins a long and gentle climb of two kilometres; then there's a steeper two kilometres to Craycroft, which winds back to Sunrise. It's quieter on Kolb, only local residents and car traffic making for the Loews resort and the parking lot for the Ventana Canyon hiking trailhead, about halfway along. DMB and Kristen have hiked that trail: a challenging climb into the foothills. Fun.

Past the light leading into the golf course the road steepens a little, and around a gentle bend there's something in the shoulder that can be spotted from fifty metres away. A dead rabbit, it turns out, up against the cement curbs; it's almost the same colour as the concrete. No squish of guts, no scattered body parts, no blood smear on the tarmac, it looks to have died without violence, as if it crossed the road, fell over from a heart attack and perished whole. Is that possible? Too bad, little buddy.

Dead rabbits, dead birds.

Up and up, then a kilometre of descent, wheee, which leads to a sudden, steep, but short climb before the plunge down to Sunrise. 40 k.p.h., 50, 60, 70, whoa, the road is dead straight and the surface perfectly smooth, but that's a lot of speed to take to the intersection and the lights. Right turn, then, and heading west again, sun higher now, a bit of sweat on the forehead. Two little rises before the drop to Swan Road and the Starbucks in the mall where DMB usually stops for latte.

At the top of the second rise another dead rabbit, this one just in the right-hand lane, scraped across the tarmac, blood smear, ugly. DMB gulps air. This is too much, now. Three little deaths in the space of ten kilometres, the passage of thirty minutes. It feels like an omen, a sign. DMB knows it isn't, he's a rationalist, a believer in science, not portents, but when he gets his latte at Starbucks he sits a little longer than usual and ponders a heart rate that isn't dropping back into the normal zone as quickly as it should be.

In the early years of the new millennium we spend a lot of time outdoors with our son, Andrew: cross-country skiing in the winter and cycling in the summer. He's a big boy, approaching six feet tall as he becomes a teenager, and like his pals, who come over to the house from time to time, an endless consumer of food. "The Pit," I call him. At suppers, he eats as much as Kristen and I combined, and neither of us is a slouch in the food department. "You could feed them cardboard," Kristen says of Andrew and his pals, "and as long as it had ketchup on it, they would be looking for seconds before you could turn your back." We ride the neighbourhood, the three of us, Kristen and I on cross-bikes we've bought, sturdy machines with hybrid tires and more compact geometry than road bikes, and Andrew on a mountain bike, initially a junior machine, and then the Proflex. That works for a year or two but as he grows, he becomes interested in road cycling, so he rides Kristen's Peloton for a season, then I buy a new road bike and he inherits my Trek 5000, a machine many an enthusiastic cyclist would be proud to own.

On weekends we put the bikes on the car and drive to Birds Hill Park, about an hour from our door. As its name suggests, it's a recreational site with recently paved roads, wide shoulders, and two or three hills—not leg-busters in the way of the sharp ascents in France, England, and Italy, but challenging enough. Like my own, Andrew's size slows him considerably on ascents: Kristen, who is sixty pounds lighter than us, recalls reading that every pound adds 20 seconds to a climb. But our greater weight serves us well on descents; the extra weight shoots us down the slopes; "gravity sledder," British cyclists quip: a rider you passed going up the hill who then passes you on the way down.

There are competitions that take place at Birds Hill Park and other places in the area and one summer Andrew enters a junior race, two laps around the inner circuit at Birds Hill, about twenty kilometres. At the start line, the organizers pin a square of cloth with a number stencilled on it to his back; they also place a retaining tag on the rear cassette of his bike: it prevents him from using the biggest gears, a measure that is supposed to keep the race's playing field level. Standing at the line, the ten juniors in Andrew's age category look nervous and focused. He starts well, using his size to muscle through the first lap in the lead. But that same size betrays him during the second lap, where stamina on the hills becomes important: he finishes third.

The folks gathered at the race's finish area chat with us while the senior racers prepare to take the stage: stretching, checking last-minute mechanicals, glugging sports drinks. A guy admiring my French-made bike says, "You should give the next race a go yourself." A woman says to Kristen, "You should join our Tuesday cycling group, women only, it's a lot of fun." We both decline. We like riding together; and we know ourselves too well. We're competitive: I was a pretty good hockey player in my day; Kristen was on her college field hockey squad. If we start to compete, we'll throw ourselves into it to the point of compulsion, and the recreational rides we do as a couple will be sacrificed. Besides, I've got a more important competition in my life: the competition *for* my life.

After the one race at Birds Hill Park, Andrew packs in competition, too. He's on the rugby team at his high school, a key player because of his height and overall size; he's the guy they throw into the air to grab the ball at the restart called "line-out." By his graduating year, he's the team captain, and at the end of the rugby season, he receives the trophy for the most important player on the squad. In the summer that follows, he's selected to the squad representing the province at the Canada Summer Games. I don't know who's more pleased: we both glow when Kristen takes a photo of the two of us, Andrew wearing his swishy Canada Games outfit.

Kristen and I bash on on the road bikes. She buys the top-end Canadian-made Cervelo to match my Time and we travel to France every summer, going over parts of stages of Le Tour: in the Pyrenees, around Montpellier, in the Bordeaux area. We go to the Okanagan in British Columbia, which turns out to be great cycling but also very expensive: the proprietor of a B&B we stay at quips: "BC stands for *bring cash*"; we revisit the Dordogne; we drive every year to Wisconsin, only seven hours by car and a cycling Valhalla, though compared to France or Italy, the food leaves a lot to be wished for.

DEAD MAN ON A BIKE:

DOWN MOUNT LEMMON

> *Get a bicycle. You will not regret it—if you live.*
> ~ Mark Twain

A slug of water, a moment to pull on the wind vest. Now it's down. "See you at the bottom," Bill says. DMB is taller than Bill but maybe not as heavy, and weight matters on the descent. Imagine every pound you carry up the mountain as a pound of butter strapped to your back. When you're ten pounds overweight, you're dragging ten blocks of butter up the mountain that you need not. No surprise, then, how obsessive the pros are about their weight. They throw off *empty* water bottles at the bases of mountains. But weight makes you go faster on the descent.

Down in the drops, then, knees pinched against the top tube, butt as far back on the saddle as possible: aerodynamics.

Forty kilometres per hour, 45, 50, 55. Gotta be careful on the bends, the g-forces drag you toward the verge and then push you across the centre yellow line; there are cars coming up the mountain. Splat. No good. Try not to touch the brakes, lean into the curve, stick out the inside knee. He could crash here: road rash, broken collarbone, fractured vertebrae. The season would be over. But you kick a few times even on a fast descent, push the bike through the bends, hold the apex of the curve, heart in mouth. One flinch, one bit of missed timing, a puncture, a rock in the road, or a broken spoke, and you're toast. Don't think of that. To be a cyclist involves a certain amount of willed stupidity. You have to be a fatalist. Let the bike go, come what will. So be it.

Quick glance at the computer: 65. This bike develops front-wheel wobble on descents, has sent him down the edge of the verge, into the toulee bushes, once straight across the tarmac in front of an oncoming car. Shiiit. Dead Man on a Bike was nearly Dead Man Not on a Bike.

Jesus, a bug-gag, some little bugger has flown into his mouth and he's swallowed it. He hacks a few times. Shoots water into his mouth. Bugs, he hates them. Filthy things all around, spread disease. He takes a long swallow of water and stifles the gag reflex. He tastes something like dirt in his mouth. Shiiit!

One curve, then another. A sign warning of a chicane-type bend. Handful of brakes. Down to 45 k.p.h., 40.

He came to cycling a little late to be a good descender. To climb you have to find a rhythm that puts the body to sleep. To descend, the mind has to go to sleep. You cannot think of the consequences, you can't think at all, you have to leave it to the body. The little fast twitches, the nerve to stay with the apex of the curve, the guts to master the g-forces tugging you toward the verge, they have to be there, they have to have been there since way back, childhood, when you rode BMX, or whatever. It helps to be an airhead.

Suddenly the road opens into the straight downhill stretch that delivers the bike to the base of the mountain. Wheee. At the bottom he glances back quickly: here comes Bill, fluorescent yellow windbreaker flapping in the wind. Okay, then, okay. Old farts with joint issues and gut problems, they'll pay for this tomorrow—but today, today they're alive in the desert, today is all that matters.

We can't live each day as if it's our last, so what can we do? There will come a day when you don't want to live anymore, when there's no fight left, nothing more to enjoy, when the cry of the crows and the first light of dawn are only reminders of the betrayal that is the body, wracked by the cancer that waits to take away our last breath. Until that day, we press on, aiming for the first sip of morning coffee, the joy of the child's day, the first push of the pedals into a misty morning, air like breath on our skin. We can linger on those moments, all the while knowing they will not last, and that final morning will come, and take us away.

One spring we're in France, going over a stage of the Tour. It's a bright, breezy morning near the Pyrenean regional town of Foix, itself situated near the lovely Ariège River in the part of France so far to the south it's almost in Spain. Indeed, some of the local names look more Spanish than French: Port de Balès. Though you wouldn't want to mention this to the locals, who are fiercely français.

We've been cruising along flattish bits of road that follow the

Ariège, pedalling easily as we prepare to climb one of the "iconic" mountain passes of the area, Col de Port, only an eleven-kilometre ascent at an average pitch of 5.5 per cent, according to the official records, but they do not take into account the "false flats" that lead to the climb proper, another five or six kilometres at the leg-taxing grade of 3 per cent. But prior to any of that there's a hill of a kilometre or so, followed by a descent of a similar distance. We're grinding up it at a relaxed pace, trying not to *blow* our legs, saving them for the real ascent ahead.

The road winds. We come around a bend and see a guy also climbing the hill a couple hundred metres ahead of us. We close the gap. And see that he's on a cross bike with its fatter tires. We can tell he's older, somewhat portly in the manner of cyclists who've been riders for most of their lives: heavy torso, "beer" belly, but fit and muscular legs. And fully kitted out: colourful jersey, bright cycling shoes. As we approach, there's a distinctive sound: brrr-up. A pungent odour wafts back towards us. We glance at each other and smirk. The gap closes to less than ten metres, *brr-up*, then five, *brru-ppp*. By this time, we're trying hard not to laugh aloud, blinking from the smell, stifling giggles. We pass. Because of the slope, it takes some seconds. *Brrr-up.* "*Bonjour,*" we call out. "*Bonjour,*" the man says in a hearty voice, though he's puffing hard, as well as sweating. And laughing. The smell that is his aura is quite strong. "Is jet propel," he calls out in English, having surmised we're not from France: "Is jet propel," he repeats, laughing as we pedal on.

One autumn we're in Italy, staying in a small town south of Florence. It's a hot afternoon, and we're returning to our *pensione* after a day of riding the hills. Sweat runs down our faces. In the past hour the water in our bottles has transformed from tepid to hot. In Tuscany you're either climbing or descending. There are very few flat stretches and they are rarely longer than a kilometre. We're on a descent, about halfway down a mildish drop of several kilometres. Kristen is ahead, leaning into the curves, I'm lost in thought as we whistle to the bottom of the descent, so lost that I do not see the sharpish bend coming, or sense its pull on the bike as g-forces assert their pressure. In a moment my front wheel is off the tarmac and seconds later the whole bike is into the gravel verge, the front wheel slewing as it plows through loose stones and sand, the rear wheel beginning to skid out. I'm going down. Shit, my shoulder will hit hard ground, I'll break my collarbone, smash my hip, bash knees and ankles, scrape my cheek. These thoughts flash through my brain as I struggle to right the bike, stones pinging on its undercarriage, my one foot grazing grasses in the ditch. Somehow, I keep it together, keep the bike upright, though it's bouncing wildly over gravel and sand as I brake and try to fight back onto the tarmac. My heart flails crazily in my chest, I've developed an instant headache. But I'm back on the tarmac, arms trembling. I've been off the road for only fifty metres or so, a matter of maybe twenty seconds. Ahead of me, Kristen has slowed, aware of something amiss. "You all right?" she asks, as I close the gap between us. "Yeah," I mutter through parched lips, "just. I went into the toulees back there."

One summer we're in Wisconsin, riding that state's wonderful side roads, roads that undulate, sweep along shallow rivers, climb sharply from the Mississippi and east into farmland, heartland America, smooth blacktop and almost no vehicle traffic, a cyclist's dreamland. Our ride has taken us out of Galesville, a town not too far from the biggest centre in the area, La Crosse. It's hot as noon approaches; we've been on the bikes for several hours, going up and down, enjoying the quiet, bucolic landscape of this forgotten corner of America. The town we're coming into is Ettrick: one gas station, one general store, a fast-food place, an implement dealership, several boarded-over and decrepit store fronts, insurance agency, and bar. We leave the bikes outside the last and go inside. The half dozen locals at the bar and around the pool table check us out as we cross from the entrance, the cleats of our shoes clicking on the wooden floor. There's a menu on a chalkboard behind the bar. We order two light beers and two hamburgers with fries, take a seat at a table, and wait for our food to arrive. Sweat drips down my nose. Kristen does a quick stretch of her arms.

"Good ride," I say.

"Great ride," Kristen responds. "It's so quiet on the roads, the countryside is empty. Just the occasional pickup, every now and then a farmer in a field."

"Yeah. A deserted landscape. I guess most of the kids head to cities. What's left behind is the residuals, these folks. The residual Cheese-Heads."

"Huh," Kristen says, "residual Badgers."

We look around. On the walls hang rifles and deer antlers.

The guys around the pool table smash the balls into each other. When they're not shooting, they prop their beer bottles on the table. They're wearing work shirts and baseball caps.

At the bar a guy is saying the marines should just go into the Middle East and sort the whole mess out, once and for all.

"That's right," the woman standing beside him says. "All that's required is a little American what-you-call."

"Diplomacy," the guy says. "Bazooka diplomacy. Drone diplomacy."

"Ingenuity, is what I was getting at."

"American-style diplomacy," the guy adds, laughing and batting one palm on the bar. He's wearing a Deere baseball cap and they both have cigarettes on their lips, puffing and blowing smoke into the air.

The woman laughs, a high-pitched snort. "We had to sort out things in Korea and even before that in Italy way back when." She glances toward us, checking if we can overhear what she's saying. We gaze back but don't say anything.

Satisfied she does, indeed, have an audience, she turns back to her companion. "You know," she goes on, "them Eye-Talians, they're a piece of work."

The guy takes a slug of his beer. "How's that, now, Gerry?"

"They claim they invented pizza." The woman puffs into the air, takes a slug of beer and sets the bottle onto the bar with a sharp crack. "Well, they did not. Pizza was invented right here in America. In New York, like."

"That so?"

"Maybe Baltimore or Boston. Somewheres in the east, like."

"That so."

The woman glances at us again. There's a half smile on her lips as she goes on. "See, them Eye-Talians, they claim they invented pizza, but all they done was add baysil and garlic and shit like that, fancy stuff, olive oil and anchovies, which I cannot personally stand, the smell, you know, but pizza itself, pizza was invented right here in the good ole US of A."

"That so, now, Gerry?"

"That there is God's own truth."

One spring we're cycling out to Headingley, Andrew, Kristen, and I. We're on Wellington Crescent a few blocks before Assiniboine Park, riding west. There's a little downhill just past the Rady Centre where we make a sharp turn down a side street that takes us to Corydon Avenue. I'm in the lead, enjoying the speed of the bike as it plunges down the hill. Too late I see that it rained in this neighbourhood in the night, there's a sheen of water on the tarmac, just the worst kind of road wetness, a thin film of runoff that mixes with the oil off cars and the tarmac's own oils to produce a slick and slippery surface. I'm going down. The bike is into the turn, I'm braking, but it's too late, the front wheel skids out, in the blink of an eye my body hits the road, I'm sliding along the tarmac, the bike flying out ahead of me and into the curb, my helmet ping-ponging on the road, one shoulder, hip, knee, and ankle, scraping and bouncing on hard ground until I too come to rest against the curb. I lie for several seconds, looking at the sky, then up into the faces of Kristen and Andrew. My heart is hammering in my throat; temples searing with headache. "I'm okay," I gasp, feeling already the pulse of blood in my shoulder and hip. "I'm okay."

One autumn we're in France, breezing about in Breton, up and down, enjoying bright and sunny weather, listening to the tires whir, chatting about the rolling terrain and wooded hills, marvelling at the road we're on, the tarmac seemingly laid the week before. We pass a giant bicycle erected from aluminum on the slope of a hill; on the road surface the words ALLEZ SCANLON, VOECKLER ALLEZ. The kilometres tick by. It's after noon and we're hot, we're tired. We approach a town. Roll down the main street, where there's a bar. We dismount and leave the bicycles outside and go into the bar, order two *pressions*, draft beer, and sit to drink. On the TV a bike race is being shown, and the men in the bar are standing in front of it watching, exchanging observations. From time to time a ripple of excitement passes through them. The race is close, two riders in a breakaway out front, the route going up and down hills much like those we've just been riding on. Suddenly the men in the bar abandon the TV as one, running out of the door onto the street, voices high in excitement. We jump up and follow them. In a moment two cyclists come over the crest we've just come down, only they're moving fast, flying, heads down, and in another moment an entire pack appears, hard on the heels of the two leaders. It's the bike race we've been watching on TV. The men from the bar shout *allez, allez*. The whole peloton whirs past, a cacophony of tires on tarmac and spokes cutting through air, brightly coloured jerseys, whoosh of wind. A hundred or more pro cyclists are past the bar in a second, disappearing at the bottom of the hill and out of town. The men retreat to the TV in the bar, pointing and laughing. We've just witnessed the passage of the GP de Plouay, one of the most prestigious one-day races in Europe.

One summer we're in Wisconsin, doing a ride in Trempealeau county called Top of the World, a wonderful climbing jaunt that leads to terrific descents at its finish. At the halfway point of the circuit we're at the words painted on the blacktop, "Top O' The World," a vista in all four directions of rural Wisconsin: cornfields to one side, woods to the other, and in the distance, Jersey cattle in a wide meadow. We drink from our water bottles as we begin the descent. Though the surface is smooth, the road winds; sometimes there are sharpish bends, and we lean into them to gather speed. Our speed goes from 30 k.p.h. to 40 and 50, and then 60. Kristen is ahead, tucking low on her machine, taking the bends with greater and greater pace. About halfway down, I sense the front wheel of my bike starting to shake a little, and within moments it's wobbling crazily, looking like it might bend into taco chip shape, the momentum of the bike shaking my arms. The bike is out of control, and when I brake, the shaking seems to get worse, it pulls the bike towards the centre of the road, and then in a flash I'm across the solid yellow line and heading toward the far side. I'm in panic mode, trying to stay upright, trying to bring the shaking bike under control. It has a mind of its own. *I'm going down, I'm going down,* broken collarbone, smashed face, edemas, the end of being on the bike for a long while. Shit. The bike flies across the tarmac and into a mowed ditch on the far side, and as it slows, I realize I'm on the front lawn of a house, a miniature wishing well to one side, garden gnomes to the other. The bike is still moving. But it's upright. So is my heart. I stand on the pedals and ride back through the ditch, then cross the road and resume the descent. Slowly. At the bottom, Kristen is waiting. "What happened?" she asks. "Shit," I gasp. I tell her how the front wheel began to wobble, how the bike shot across the road into the far ditch. "Jesus," she says, "you were lucky there were no cars." It's a thought I had not had. If a car had been coming from the opposite direction—even the same direction as we were headed—I would have been struck, probably killed. We sip from our water bottles. "Jesus," I say. My arms are trembling, sweat is pouring from my brow. We pedal on.

In Italy one summer we're sitting at a bar drinking caffè with our Italian friend, Mario. He's driven to the town of Gaiole to meet us for lunch. We're on our way back from Montalcino, riding north to the town Mario comes from, near Florence. I'm telling him about Lance Armstrong, telling him about my suspicions that he's been taking drugs for years, that he would not have won the Tour de France without the drugs. "One day," I say, "he's going to be exposed, one day the whole world will know he's a cheat." "Forget about it," he says, "they'll never expose him." "No," I insist, "you're wrong, Americans are Puritans, they believe in right and wrong, in black and white." "Yes," he counters, "but Americans don't run the Tour, the Tour is run by the French, and like Italians, they know it's better for them he not be exposed, even if he's a cheat. If they expose him now, after he's won all those Tours, it's bad for him but it's much worse for them, it casts a black shadow over the whole sport, it scares away sponsors, it brings the famous Tour into disrepute. Millions are lost, and money is what the Tour is all about, money is what everything is all about—in the end. You see." He sips his caffè; I sip mine. I have to admit: he has a point.

One autumn we're in France, staying near the college town of Cahors in the Dordogne, riding the back roads. The Dordogne is a famous region of France; much of the Hundred Years War was contested in the area. It's dotted with striking castles and their battlements—Biron, Bonaguil—and numerous fortresses on the summits of hills. We've just climbed one of those hills, though not to a famous *bastide*, and I'm off my bike and on the grass near a gravel road, lying on my side in the fetal position, rocking back and forth, my hands clenched over my gut. I feel like vomiting, but I'm not vomiting, I'm in the midst of one of the attacks that strike me from time to time, something to do with the cancer. If I could vomit, I might well feel better, but that's out of the question. What I can do is lie on my side, breathe deeply, and rock back and forth until the clenching—cramps—passes. Kristen sits beside me on the grass, one hand on my shoulder, fingers lightly stroking one temple. "Oh Jesus," I moan between clenched teeth, "oh Christ." Birds are twittering in the bushes nearby, cars go by on the road. The sky is blue with fluffy white clouds, a *Simpsons* sky. We both know the attack will pass. In five minutes, ten, fifteen, I will be able to roll onto my back, stretch out the muscles in my gut; in another ten minutes, the pain will ease, and then I will sit and sip water, eventually climb back on the bike, pedal on. I'll have a grainy headache and my guts will hurt for a few hours. The day's ride will not be ruined, though there will be a shadow over it; life will go on.

One spring we're in the south of England. At the end of a day's riding we've retired to the bar at our hotel, having a beer and a plate of food. It's "rump roast night" at the hotel, something of a tradition in the area, the hotel bars taking turns every Friday night at serving up complete suppers for five pounds. The rump roast is well done and resembles the proverbial shoe leather. It's accompanied by chips, peas, and broccoli. Washed down with a pint, it's hearty rural fare; you leave with a full belly, and at five pounds it's a good deal. Not good dining, but a good deal.

Our seats are at a table that's just close enough to the bar proper for us to overhear what's going on up there. One of the local wags is holding court. "Last week," he's saying, "last Friday it was me and Toby after work in here and he says to me, he says, they're doing the rump roast over to Stockbridge tonight, we should hop in the car and drive over, a couple of bachelors, us, they got a couple of them there Pakis running the Bell now, wearing them *turbos*, you know, all knotted around their heads, a couple of them *turbos*, and they're throwing in the first pint free. Yeah, says I, a good idear but we're pretty much laggered up by then and we run the risk of DUI, it's hardly worth it, when you're laggered up and the filth nab you, you lose the tags for three months. No worry, Toby says, I got the layoff notice today so I'll drive your car and if we get stopped you can pay the fine, you still having the pay cheque coming in, and I'll take the other, I'll be on the dole anyways, I won't be needing to drive anywhere." The guy with him is chuckling, as is the bartender as he pours the wag another pint. He takes a slug of it and looks around to see if he has an audience. The couple beside him at the bar are engaged in an intense exchange, but a second couple at a nearby table are looking his way, as are we. The wag glances up at the TV behind the bar: a clip of Prince Charles and Diana smiling into the cameras. "Now there," the wag's buddy says, "is one lucky guy, he's not worrying about the boss Monday mornings or making the car payment." "Too right," the wag says, "but that Toby, now, he says, it's a godawful thing being a royal, you gotta bust your butt out to all these functions and groundbreakings and whatnot and smile for the camera, and I says, what, you kidding me, it's a lark, it's a doggle, flying around in a private jet, eating posh meals, wearing fancy clothes, and that Charles, if he weren't a royal, a prince, you think he'd be getting it off with a pretty little thing like Diana, he's one lucky duck, that one, and when I say duck I mean *horse*, you seen that face, a face only a mother could love, except I'm not so sure she does, if you go by what's in the papers, she should be handing over the crown to him by now, but she's hanging onto that thing like it's a life preserver, I'm not so sure everything is just hunky-dory between that horsey old lot at Windsor Castle, like." He's laughing himself, now, glancing around and catching our eyes, tipping his pint at us. He's a performer, the local entertainment on a Friday night. He takes another slug of beer and turns back to his mate. "Now what was I just saying there, Jerry?"

DEAD MAN ON A BIKE:

DMB TAKES DRUGS

Every man dies ... not every man really lives.
~ William Ross Wallace

Lutetium 177, a radioisotope "smart bomb" designed to attack cancer cells and reduce tumour growth, maybe reduce tumour mass itself. Powerful stuff, it knocks him sideways for at least a week, pounds the immune system, cuts into bone marrow. There is excruciating pain—in the back, in the legs, in the shoulders: wherever the body is weak or can be easily attacked; pain that only can be dealt with by doses of steroids and handfuls of Tylenol 3. There are sleepless nights—and drugs to deal with that: tranquillizers, anti-inflammatories, sleeping potions. Then come the side effects, including glorious constipation. You don't want to go there.

DMB is on the bike for the first time since the treatment, exactly one week later. A pleasant day on the prairies, sunny, warm, the south wind blowing up from America with the promise of summer. He cannot escape metaphor.

Thatcher Drive, a lovely flattish stretch that runs along the Red River to the south of the city. Good to be out: the whirr of wheels, heart thumping in the chest, breeze fresh on the face. Ah, the twitter of red-winged blackbirds, sitting in the bulrushes, a piercing crackling whistle. I salute you, blackbirds, he thinks.

Here's a cyclist coming from the other direction: tip of the hand. Why is it the guy wearing the goofiest helmet always has the ready wave and the guy kitted out in team colours has no time for other cyclists?

Now a meadowlark calls. He glances up. Sitting on a telephone wire. Sing, my friend.

Just past the halfway point, a dead deer on the opposite side of the road, white belly, black nose, a recent killing; the crows have not got to it yet, though flies are buzzing round. Shit, DMB thinks; this is not metaphor. "Peace to your ashes," he mutters under his breath, "peace to your bones."

Do not let this ruin the ride. His mantra.

Which do we fear more, death or dying? Process or state? When Gogol screamed out, was it because his mind was terrified by the thought of no longer being sentient, or was the body in such excruciating pain that there was no other response? Some people really do *fear* death, he's read, some wake in the night calling out *No, No, No,* the terror is that real. Has he felt that? No.

Oh, this is hard, the legs are tired, energy is low. His red blood cell count is down these days, the body working hard to get oxygen; platelets down, white blood cells, the body is working at about 50 per cent, his reliable old friend, though it all rebounds (sort of) in a few weeks. But right now his body is beat. This is not a hard ride but this is a hard ride.

Keep going. That's the ticket. Put the head down into the wind, feel the muscles built up in Tucson over the past months. Heart rate: 137. Not too high. But shit, the wind. The weather guesstimators said south 20 k.p.h., but this is more like 30. Curse their hopeless bones. Still, out here, doing it.

Death or dying. You must be in one camp or the other. He can't place himself, but he gives it a long thought. It will be okay, he thinks, not to be here. From time to time he meditates, zones into a somewhere else that he cannot describe—no one can. But you can get there. That's *not being here,* at least in one way. He believes he can accept that: Death. Dying, then? Is it feeling the cold hand of Death on the shoulder, the accompanying pains—well, today with all the meds more anguish than pain, the anguish of passing. *Don't let me go!* Is that what he'll say at the final moment? Or will he understand the moment, acknowledge it, say *I'm already dead*?

Here's the deer again, on the return. Crikey. But at least the wind is behind him now, he's torquing along, 30 k.p.h., 32, 35. Okay, this is good. The riding is good, the ride is what it's all about. Relax and let go, blink away those dark thoughts. He'll figure out the Death and Dying bit later.

One year blends into the next. Through the last decade of the twentieth century and into the opening years of the new millennium, we travel to Mexico every winter, two and three weeks in the sun, away from the prairie winter: its frigid temperatures and howling winds and snow. Away from being a cancer patient. We take the bikes with us and do a ride every morning, up with the sun to complete a fifty-kilometre circuit before the sun rises over the palm trees and beats its unrelenting tattoo. But one year I develop stomach sickness while down there and spend two days in bed, sweating and hallucinating. The next year the gut sickness hits me on the flight home. I see my physician, tell him the story. "This is not unusual, gut problems in Mexico," he tells me as he writes up a prescription for antibiotic, "but with you it's a bit more serious; your immune system is pretty fragile. You really should not be travelling there."

In the summer we're deep in conversation about whether or not to return to Mexico: it's an important break in our everyday lives. Kristen gets away from her demanding work, I can forget about cancer for a few weeks. But on the other side, there's the gut stuff. We want to ride the bikes, we have to ride; the question now is: where?

At the bike store I tell Scot that we've spent a long weekend in Phoenix, where we rented bicycles and enjoyed riding in the desert heat. "Phoenix is good," he says, "but Tucson is better; that's the place to go. Every cyclist I've known who's been there can't stop talking about it; great hills to climb, great roads, great climate; a lot of pro teams train there in winter." I consult a site called Vacationhomes and we rent a condo for ten days the following November. Heat, sun, wonderful roads, fantastic mountain and desert riding, great Mexican restaurants and, in comparison with the resort in Mexico, cheap. We can vacation for a month in Tucson at the same cost as a week in Mexico. We're determined to go back.

In the spring of 2008 we pack up the bikes and take them south with us. We like the city immensely. Younger brother to bustling Phoenix, a hundred miles down the road, it's more laid back, less concrete and freeways, packed with cyclists and good cycling roads, and in brief, more like Winnipeg. After a month of cycling and eating Mexican food, we're sold. We make plans to come back in six months. There's only one problem: schlepping the bikes through the airports is time-consuming, costly, a nuisance. Why not leave them in Arizona and ride the new ones we're planning on buying at home? We approach the owner of a Tucson bike shop. "Sure," Mac says, "I'll store them for you and tune them up for when you come back in November: a hundred bucks." Deal. We develop a routine: five weeks of sun in November and December; six weeks in March and April. The woman who rents us the condo says, "We have a standing arrangement; the place is yours, as long as you let me know in advance." We become snowbirds.

DEAD MAN ON A BIKE:

TUCSON PAEAN II

When I see an adult on a bicycle, I do not despair
about the future of the human race.
~ H.G. Wells

A ride around the foot of Mount Lemmon. No going up there today. The last time the sacroiliac popped out of joint, the sciatic nerve was pinched, days of pain and nights of no sleep. DMB had to go to the chiropractor, hit the Celebrex for a few days. So none of that today.

Instead a loop down Catalina Highway north, then a swing east before heading down Soldier Trail, south, before returning to Catalina Highway on Tanque Verde, a nice ride, around twenty-five kilometres, takes about an hour. He'll do two laps.

Catalina Highway climbs from Tanque Verde to the foot of Mount Lemmon. To the naked eye the ride looks flat, but it's a continuous gentle climb, a false flat at about 3 per cent, slows you down. He watches the bike's speed drop from 27 to 25 to 22, and then 18. Cyclists coming off Mount Lemmon from the other direction tip their heads from the far side of the highway, raise hands in greeting, whip past on the long gentle descent into the city. DMB thinks: I salute you, climbers; I envy your strong bodies. In eight kilometres he hits the base of Mount Lemmon and makes the turn east away from the ascent. It hurts a bit not to be making the climb; but it would hurt a lot more to make it.

Soldier Trail is a bit rough in places, the bike jumps about on the tarmac, his wrists and elbows feel the lumpiness of the road. No problem. The sun beats down, sweat on the brow, a nice long pull, it's all good. He's out here.

Up ahead on the verge there's an animal. He didn't see it at first.

93

It stands motionless. It looks like a dog but as he comes closer he sees its markings are those of a coyote. Its eyes are studying him but it hasn't moved since he caught sight of it, tail curled into a question mark. Then it lowers its head as if to attack. An instant of panic in his chest. Rabid dogs have been known to attack cyclists, sink their teeth into shins. His season of cycling is in jeopardy: hospital, antibiotics. Why does the coyote just stand there, gazing at him?

He keeps the pedals turning but he's ready to jump off the bike and use it to defend himself. When he's twenty metres away, the coyote suddenly lifts its nose, sniffs the air, and then turns and darts down into the ditch. DMB passes. He looks into the ditch. No sign of it. Good thinking, buddy.

His heart rate is high now, and not just from the climb. The hands are back on the hoods, resting. The guy with the yellow wristbands won't use flat bars, so none of the American kids do either. The guy in the yellow bands fast-pedals in easy gears so all the American kids do too. Piss on them.

It's a crappy attitude, he realizes it. What grudge does he have with the famous cyclist? So he's likely a cheat—who isn't in that world? He's a bastard, probably, too, but he's done some good things for recovering cancer patients. Live and let live. He's a bastard but not the worst kind of bastard. Maybe. In any case, DMB wears the yellow band; has never taken it off since he first put it on: how many years now—eight? He bought a box from the foundation and doled them out to friends.

A sharp ascent of no more than two hundred metres, a fast plunge down, fifty metres of flat, then repeat. Wheee. Cycling. A few moments of grinding up a hill, then the thrill of the reckless descent on bumpy tarmac into a sharpish bend at the bottom of a hill where you have to brake suddenly at a stop sign or go flying through an intersection, risking death, wild and crazy stuff, heads up for cars turning onto Soldier, putting life on the line in a minor way, life is always on the line. Does it get any better than this?

The next ride will be better. Is the next ride always better?

Sitting in restaurants in France, overhearing the conversations at nearby tables, you notice an intriguing phenomenon: when French diners are not discussing the food they are currently eating, they're conferring about the food they will soon be eating, relishing recollections of meals past. Lunch tomorrow awaits; supper, come Saturday night, beckons. Life for them is one prolonged feast, part of their *joie de vivre*, and though this meal is grand, the next meal promises to be even more grand. Oysters, perhaps, duck *confit*, *cassoulet*, *coq au vin*, *grenadins de veau*—and don't forget the wine! Or the cheese. Or the *crème brulée*.

For cyclists much the same applies. A different kind of moveable feast, more moveable, but a grand indulgence. You have just climbed one of the iconic cols—or one of the not so famous—or swept through the hills of a delightful region, or skirted the Mississippi. But tomorrow crooks its enticing finger. You put away the bikes; you down a cold beer; you wash up and change into "civvies"; you down another cold beer. "Boy, that sure hits the spot." You're on the floor in a hotel room, stretching: don't forget the hip lunge that Tim, the chiro, taught you: tall, tall, tall. Feels good. You turn to your cycling companion: "What you got in mind for tomorrow?" That stretch along the Oust River beckons; or the climb out of the Columbia valley; the Col du Vent; Dunham to Frelighsburg—the apples are ripe just now, we can stop and eat galas fresh off the tree. Today was sweet, very sweet, but tomorrow promises to be even sweeter, you can taste it like those apples—crisp to the tooth, juicy on the lips.

The Great River Ride runs from Prescott in Wisconsin to Dubuque, Iowa. The best part is found from Prescott to just past Fountain City along the Mississippi in Wisconsin. Highway 35 on the road map. About 135 kilometres in length, it winds and sweeps its course through eleven towns that once were centres of commerce on the great river: fishing villages and ports of call in the days when transportation meant travel on water routes. Some of them are still active hubs of commerce. But now most of those towns are home to B&Bs, to camping grounds, knickknack stores, modest restaurants, and tourist information centres.

We're on our road bikes pedalling south, having put the most challenging section of the route—between Prescott and Bay City—behind us. That was sharply undulant hills, one following hard on the heels of another, perhaps twenty climbs in all. That was sweat on the brow, standing up on the pedals, and heart rates in the red zone. Jagged rock outcroppings on the eastern flank, "bluffs," they're called here, and tall pines occasionally giving way to delightful views of the winking Mississippi on the western flank.

It's a lovely day, mid morning, and the sky above is a mix of fluffy white clouds and giant blue patches. Hawks float overhead. Flurries of small birds dart from one side of the road to the other. A skunk wobbled along the verge on the bluff side some kilometres back. Riding in the lead, I called out to Kristen: "Whoa!" She laughed: "Is Pepé le Pew." The stands of heady-smelling pines are foregrounded by shrubs with bright yellow flowers and tall grasses that wave gently in the slight breeze from the north.

Wisconsin is a great place to cycle. The travel brochures say so, but they always claim that, even about the Eastern Townships of Quebec, where you take your life in your hands on narrow and busy roads where lorries steam past frequently, seemingly intent on brushing you into the ditch. The Wisconsin terrain is very inviting: rolling hills, silent forests, the great river itself. Roads are well maintained and quiet. They undulate. You look ahead and see the gentle sweep of a curve, and when you are at its apex, glimpse a rise in the distance, the kind of challenging, steep, sharp but brief ascent that you came to ride.

Just out of Bay City we begin just such a rise. It's gentle at first, but after several hundred metres begins to steepen. We gear down. Our hearts speed up as the wheels of our bikes slow. Ahead of me, Kristen stands for a half minute to bring different muscles into play. Her puffing is audible. This climb is what cycling magazines call *moderate to strenuous*. We change chain rings and work the lower gears. Kristen drops back for a moment and says, "This is a good one." We push on, the only sounds our breathing and the ticking of pedals under feet. In five minutes we're at the summit of the 100 metres of vertical rise, where there's a pull-over and a historic marker. We read the inscription and take a snapshot. Drink water. Far below the wide river twinkles in the sunlight: it's so wide at points, three or four kilometres, that its course forms bays, and from the shore it appears to be a lake. A train line runs along the riverbed and every few minutes you hear the screeing and scrawing of iron on iron. On the river a barge we cannot see hoots and its sound echoes along the water.

It would be lovely to picnic here: the big sky, the sparkling water, the silent forest.

The descent is magnificent. The bikes pick up speed almost immediately but this is not the harrowing descent of a Tour de France col: speeds of 70+ k.p.h., white-knuckle bends whose g-forces try to suck you off the tarmac and over the precipice. This is pleasurable scooting, tires whirring, wind whistling through helmets at 45 k.p.h. Exhilarating but not frightening. The sweat we developed on the ascent cools on the descent. Heart rates drop. Ahead of me, Kristen goes deep into the drops, leans into a long curve, and when I catch up, grins broadly. "You're having fun," I say. "Believe it," she responds.

Almost before we know it we're in Maiden Rock, ten kilometres from Bay City, and soon enough another six or eight kilometres zip by and we've come to Stockholm, population 971. We chuckle at the road sign announcing the town. "I'm keeping out an eye for Helsinki," Kristen quips. We pull over at a cozy-looking restaurant, Gelly's. Inside it's crowded with locals, three women sitting at a table, four tables of guys in baseball caps and work shirts. The middle-aged waitress tells us the soups of the day are chicken rice and corn chowder. We decide on one of each and a plate of french fries. Two root beers.

Wisconsin is known as the Dairy State, and it's true you can get tangy cheddar cheese and a Devon-style cream anywhere. And "cheese curds," which seem to exist nowhere else: bits of cheddar deep fried. But the state could equally be known for root beer, which in Wisconsin is oaky with hints of vanilla and a delight-ful sharpness on the palate. No, it's not vintage wine, but it's a lovely drink, especially on a hot afternoon along the Great River Ride. Frosty mugs, frothy brew.

As I stand to leave, there's a hitch in my movement. A bit of tightness in my lower back has developed over the past days. "You look like you could use a massage," one of the nearby women calls out in a smoker's voice. Her two friends laugh aloud. They're middle-aged gals having a pleasant outing together. "Or some of your horse liniment, Elaine," her friend says. They laugh. "Sounds good," I say. "You offering the massage?" Elaine wags her finger at me. Laughter echoes in the room as the door swings shut behind us.

Stockholm gives way to Pepin and Nelson, both ribbon villages where the business places are on the main drag running through town. Brick houses sit up the hillside where the town burghers once lived, clapboard fronts in bright blues and reds closer to the river; they could be the set of a certain kind of small-town America movie. The Stars and Stripes flying from businesses and the porches of residences. Gas stations, banks, what once would have been called general stores. We eye a free-standing kiosk, about three metres square, "Grabba Java" written in red paint on its white walls. These are a phenomenon we've seen only in the USA. Tiny drive-up stands where coffee is offered for sale through a little sliding window operated by the salesperson inside. You can get a "shot," what at a more conventional bar like Starbucks would be called an espresso. We're tempted but keep moving. It's early in the afternoon, the heat of the day. Caffeine dehydrates and we're in for a fair share of that without a "shot."

Soon we're moving along at a good pace. As the Great River Ride moves south and east it also becomes flatter. The locals call this area of the state the "coulee region" because of its many valleys, the biggest being the Mississippi itself. Our speed goes from 20 k.p.h. to 25 and soon 30. There are rises and even hills, but mostly the riding between Maiden Rock and Alma is flattish, gentle, pleasant. The surface is very good. Americans take care of their roads: smooth surfaces, wide shoulders. This one is remarkably quiet: only the occasional car or pickup truck. From time to time there are stretches where the Big Muddy sparkles between stands of trees. In the distance across on its far shore there's a ridge covered with dark trees. Barges ply up and down its wide girth. Crows call out raucously from the treetops. Along the flat stretches there are farms—grain, cattle, fields of corn. Tractors stir up the dust, pickup trucks go up and down the side roads. Orchards are farther to the east. The big town of La Crosse is to the south.

The heat is bringing sweat to our arms and necks. We've zipped open our jerseys. There's little breeze on the flats and the mercury is nudging 30C. We tip back our water bottles often.

At Cochrane I consult my cyclo-computer. We've covered ninety kilometres in three and half hours. Fountain City, our destination, is about twenty-five further along the road. Another hour then. An hour of gentle curves and easy slopes where we ride side by side for brief stretches, chatting. "See that badger?" Kristen asks. It was back down the road about a kilometre, scuttling into the grass when we swished past. There was a bald eagle, too, soaring over the mighty river. The road all the way has been quiet, a few cars zipping between towns, but no diesel-belching lorries crowding the road. Motorcycles, though, which whiz past, sometimes in groups of half a dozen. One or two cyclists. Waves from across the tarmac. A lone woman sporting a bright blue and green jersey, two guys with backpacks on mountain bikes.

When we come into Fountain City we've done 114 kilometres from Bay City. It's another town that looks to be more at home in the nineteenth century than the twenty-first: wide streets, ageing buildings, a warehouse town, Kristen calls it. If you close your eyes you can almost hear the clatter of horses' hooves on the side streets. We're hot and tired and we're glad to dismount and do a little stretching on a rectangle of grass in the centre of town. "Great ride," Kristen says. "Beauty," I respond. We drain our water bottles. The two cold beers we order at a roadside bar are just the thing to cut the last of our thirst.

The bumph on the Internet claims, "The Great River Ride provides gorgeous Mississippi scenery, some of the best in the country." We think they've got that right.

Cancer changes things. Cancer changes everything. In the years immediately following diagnosis, we become more aware of how we live on a day-to-day basis: sleeping habits, diet, alcohol consumption, late-night carousing, exercise; in brief, what is going into and coming out of our bodies. All of the central moments in an ordinary day on the planet assert their consequence, things we've taken for granted for decades, never thought much about—if at all—the givens of the waking hours become rather suddenly foremost in our minds. Surprised by mortality, we question all of our habits; we become conscious of their roles in the ups and downs of our immune systems, mine especially; we learn about vitamin and mineral supplements; we go for massage therapy; consult with naturopaths. Where we once thought the "unexamined life" applied to metaphysical issues only, we see that there are other territories to go over with a critical fine-tooth comb; not just metaphysics but bodily physics: receptors and plasma and peptides and a whole host of cellular functions we did not know about previously and which did not figure into our daily concerns. We devise regimes to avoid toxins and develop programs to promote well being. Our consciousness of a whole panoply of behavioural pitfalls makes us careful about abuse as well as making us advocates of *health*. We become boring to our friends.

Other things follow. We become conscious of the brevity of time and of the necessity of doing now the things we enjoy doing, of not putting off until tomorrow, next week, the coming summer, or "retirement," the pleasures of this limited and blessed existence. We've been slapped in the face by *carpe diem* and we've come out somewhat bloodied and dazed, but also determined to make the most of time. Life—mere living—now truly seems a blessing bestowed from above. Our focus changes. Where we'd been drifting along, as most of us do, we've been given the celebrated wake-up call. In effect, we've had focus thrust upon us: life is too short to meander through it, to assume there will always be a tomorrow when we'll be able to do the things we've mused about doing but never quite felt compelled to organize ourselves to get on with. We've been strolling through the woods whistling a blithe tune, unaware of the avalanche rumbling down the nearby mountain.

One net effect is this: in the early years of the new millennium we begin to travel more. Where we were content to go on cycling trips once every year or so, we now pack up the bikes and make the transatlantic flight every year—and complement it with a North American jaunt: a spring trip and an autumn trip. When we're not cycling in the Okanagan or the Eastern Townships, we're planning to go over stages of the Tour de France, or ride the hills of Tuscany.

A shadow looms overhead. We're not anxious about mortality, nor are we frantically trying to cram as much experience as possible into our days together, but we're living in the now. And it's exhilarating. More than a little aware that this life is not a rehearsal for another yet to come, we set our eyes on the present. We buy a second set of high-end road bikes to ride in Tucson. Our friends and family maybe consider our frequent vacations and swishy bikes a bit mad. At moments we do. But we've looked into the abyss. Many do who are given the cancer death sentence—the shiver down the spine that comes with "terminal" and "two to five years"—but we feel fortunate that ours is more a life sentence, so we've come to think about pricey bikes and frequent transatlantic flights, the hell with it. *I'm only going around once* becomes a mantra. And though not fearful of the future, we're determined not to waste a day of the present.

Paradoxically, our determination to not waste time makes us more open to doing exactly that—to "waste" money on expensive wine, high-performance cars, European vacations, and high-end bicycles: all of which also, in their own way, "waste" time. We push back with this logic: cycling is something we can do together as a couple, something we enjoy doing together, and it's both a source of pleasure and healthful: vigorous but not enervating exercise. We repeat the quip of the Zen master who said, *I ride my bicycle to ride my bicycle*; it's a telling sentiment; but with us it goes a step farther: we ride our bicycles to enjoy a shared together.

DEAD MAN ON A BIKE:

ONE LOOP, THEN ANOTHER

A bicycle is a flight from sadness.
~ James E. Starrs

Birds Hill Park, a circuit—doing the outside loop—of fourteen kilometres, three gentle slopes to climb. He's riding behind Kristen, drafting on a warm Saturday morning, 18C, north wind at 15 k.p.h. Tires whir on the asphalt, wind whistles in the helmet.

This is a good ride. They're on the paved shoulder, there are few cars on the road. Above, a blue sky with fluffy thin clouds. Kristen is in the drops, he's behind and slightly left, the wind out of the north. DMB is feeling pretty good: the last radioisotope treatment was seven weeks ago, his strength has returned, wind, stamina. But another treatment looms. Forget about that.

Birds Hill is a big park, a provincial park about twenty-five kilometres east and north of the city, a park set on a ridge, just at the edge of the boreal forest—pine trees dotted amongst poplars and scrub, prairie wildflowers dotting the verge—a park that features a number of undulations. Pollen floats in the air, white scantlings from the poplars—terrible for folks with allergies.

They pass a couple on mountain bikes. *Mornin'. Mornin'.*

Here's the descent to the park's west gate: 35 k.p.h., 40, 45, 50 at the bottom, then a hairpin, slowing to check traffic coming past the gatehouse, then the start of a long but gentle climb from the west gate toward the south. Kristen is up on the pedals, attacking the climb. He follows suit. Heart rate jumps. You can do muscle tension training here, pushing a big gear while keeping the cadence under 60. Training for climbing mountains.

Where the landscape opens in front of them, about halfway along the route south, a flock of Canada geese are feeding in meadow grasses in the verge. Maybe fifty, some fledglings, little more than puffballs at this time of year. These guys have proliferated in the past decade or two. The road is dotted with greenish blobs, goose poop, these guys really can lay on the crap.

He dodges through the blobs, comes up beside Kristen, laughing. She gives him a look: what? Then she laughs too. A stringy greenish patty is trapped in the brake housing of her front wheel.

"You'll have to pick that off of there," DMB says, grinning wickedly.

"I was hoping you would—*would do me a solid.*"

"No shit," he says. "A solid."

"Straight shit."

Here's the second of the long gentle climbs, about two kilometres at maybe 3 per cent gradient. Coming towards them on the opposite side of the road are three guys on time trial bikes, doing the inside loop, where all the turns are right-handed, no need to cross traffic, perfect for time-trial riding. The loop that way is about eleven kilometres. Nods from both sides of the road as they pass.

Of course another treatment is coming next week, it will knock him sideways for ten days, maybe longer; it will be a month at least before he's back to 100 per cent, whatever that means, the 100 per cent he has in recent years become, maybe 60 per cent of what he was only a few years ago. In any case, back to the way he feels today. He sighs. It's the price you pay. Forget it for now.

Coasting downhill, then, towards the east gate, completion of the lap. He checks the computer: 31:23. A good lap. Life is a loop. Around, and then around again, the eternal return, as one philosopher put it. It's not a bad thing; it's a good thing. One circuit on a ride giving way to another; one generation looping into the next. All good.

Up the little ascent to the flat near the parking lot. Kristen has raised the pace. Maybe this lap will come in under thirty minutes.

The opposite of why me? is The Miracle: the belief/hope in sudden reversals in nature's order that transform Bad into Good in one unpredictable and unprecedented turn of fortune's wheel and rescue Fate. Such events are documented. I was raised in a church-going family and know all those magical stories—Yahweh speaking out at the last moment to Abraham, instructing him to withhold his hand; water into wine at the wedding. What sudden and awe-inspiring reversals. I have no doubt that recently diagnosed cancer patients go to bed praying for one for themselves. Who can blame them?

They happen. A woman diagnosed with breast cancer resolved to forego surgery and chemotherapy and all the other procedures of modern medicine and eat only broccoli, which contains a high concentration of the antioxidant sulforaphane. She survived, she cured herself. Miraculous. A young man whose skin was covered with hive-like tumours was told he would die if he did not have chemotherapy on a Monday. He had practised meditation for some years. From Friday night to Sunday night he meditated, using visual-imaging techniques, the way athletes do in preparation for a test. On Monday morning his tumours were gone. Miracles happen. Lazarus rises from the dead; five fishes and two loaves feed a crowd.

I'm of a more scientific bent. In my teens I gave up on the Biblical stories of my childhood, inspiring as they had been; I gave up on the biggest miracle of all: Jesus rising from the dead and ascending into heaven. Exposure to books, in particular books like *The Rise and Fall of the Third Reich* and *L'Etranger*, turned me into a skeptic. No more miracles for Wayne.

But there are scientific miracles, too: a mind-bending paradox. Miracle cures. There must have been thousands who were on the cusp between life and death when penicillin was first widely used during World War II to treat amputation infections and then released into the general population, where it proved effective against various kinds of infectious diseases (*flu*). They were saved by the drug; a scientific miracle.

People say to me: maybe a miracle drug will be discovered. Maybe. My skeptical modern mind refuses to go there. It would be equivalent to winning the lottery. And something in me won't allow for that tantalizing yet reckless kind of hope. I cannot risk it.

I've discovered, in any case, that miracle cures are not "out there," but right in front of our faces, if we open our eyes to them. In the people close at hand, the doctors and nurses who administer procedures, the massage therapist who lets you talk and blub out your fears, the wife who always listens and rarely corrects. We tend to think—is this the influence of TV?—that the thing that can save us awaits out there, but miracles reside in people, the transformative thing is right there in front of us— sometimes it is our own selves.

Meditating; practising the Zen of menial tasks; embracing love where we find it; riding a bicycle.

"Look," I say, tracing one finger along the map where a winding road runs from Saint-Martins-de-Londre to Saint-Guilhem-le-désert in the Montepellier region of France.

"Ah," Kristen says, "we've been over this route before."

"Yeah. Great ride."

"There's those gorges once you pass Le Frouzet and that wicked descent off the gorge peak down to the river."

"Gorgeous gorges."

"Har."

"The Hérault River."

"Right. I love that descent. Wide road, freshly laid tarmac."

"Don't forget the descent into Saint-Guilhem."

"I'll never forget that descent. That descent is always in my mind. My absolute fave."

I like going over the same routes we've ridden before. From the safety point of view, you know what's coming—that gravel stretch at the bottom of a descent, just where it bends sharply—watch out! But vastly more important than safety is the joy of reliving earlier moments of wonder: that breathtaking view of the river through the pines. When I was young, I went for novelty: what can we do that we haven't done before, where does that inviting road go, shouldn't we attempt the iconic climb? But now I equally like going over the same route, retracing steps, feeling the wonder of re-engagement, a stunning landscape, or a village with a notable cathedral, a town where they serve perfect *caffè* or *huîtres*. Come to think of it, I feel that way about sex, too. Going over the same ground can be marvellous. There's always a new wrinkle to an old dish: the way the osso bucco tastes slightly different this time out—which was the transformative ingredient? Saffron, anchovies? There's pleasure in repetition; in fact, Freud put his finger on this when he coined the term *repetition compulsion*. We want to repeat. Let's do that again, the Italians say with gusto: *facciamolo du nuovo.* Repetition, some may feel, breeds contempt; but for me it breeds content, content fast transforming into rapture.

Each bike ride is, in one way, the repetition of every bike ride. You clip into the pedals, jump onto the saddle, and start the wheels spinning. You feel the pull of the quads, fingers gripping handlebars, snap of your ankles as you push down and through the pedal stroke. Muscles are saying, We've done this, we enjoy this; the back curves into its familiar tuck; eyes and ears are scanning for danger ahead and behind. The entire body rises up. The experience fast becomes one of those "whole is greater than the sum of the parts" things: more than any one element, it's the entire experience that is important, the *cyclisme*, as the French say; you've re-entered the zone of the ride. It's where you want to be and how you want to live. It's your *raison d'être*.

DEAD MAN ON A BIKE:

GATES PASS

I ride my bicycle to ride my bicycle.
~ Zen proverb

On the west side of Tucson, Gates Pass, a wicked little climb of 3.5 kilometres, right at the last about 400 metres at 10–12 per cent. Heart rate shoots up, the hips are not happy, lungs burn. Then the descent, *wheee*, longer than the ascent but not quite as steep, at the bottom turning into a gentle slope, kilometre after kilometre.

He's riding with Kristen, who climbs better than him, so she gets to the peak of Gates Pass a few metres before him, but he swishes past on the descent, greater body weight by sixty pounds, mostly the reason she climbs better (he tells himself).

A hot day in the desert. Hawks swoop on the air currents, crows peck in the gravel at the side of the road. They must be the most common creature on the face of the earth. Everywhere you look, another crow: barking from a telephone line, hopping in the verge of the road. Eat anything, they will. Great mimics, too. North of Winnipeg there was once a road crew that was blasting through rock face for a few weeks. Crows gathered to poach leftovers from their lunches. At the end of two weeks, when the road crew stopped for lunch they heard the crows barking "boom, boom." Is this an apocryphal story?

Through Saguaro Park, the road still descending. They'll have to climb all this on the return. And out onto Sandario Road, a straightaway that runs toward Twin Peaks, kilometre after kilometre. Sun beats down, sweat runs to the end of the nose, drops onto the top tube. Keep pedalling, drink tepid water. Here's an animal squashed on the road so badly it's hard to tell what it was—bird, squirrel, rabbit? The wince. It's not hard to see in these little deaths his own. And then there's a wooden cross in the verge, with wilting flowers, homemade memorial. This is too much on one ride. Best not thought about.

The return ride is all uphill, much at gentle inclines, some at fairly steep. Hot head. Stop for water back in Saguaro Park at the Information Centre. More climbing, and then more under the blazing afternoon sun. This is fun? It's good to be out here. The road surface is great, the swooping hawks interesting, mountains in the distance easy on the eye. Cactus. How many kinds are there? Those giant saguaros could be a couple hundred years old.

Here's the foot of Gates Pass. Stand for thirty or fifty strokes, bring different muscles into play before doing the ascent. Now the sweat is running freely down the cheeks. One droplet, then another slides down the dark glasses, blurring vision. One more kilometre to go. A cold beer at that place about five kilometres beyond Gates Pass keeps the legs going round and round. Maybe a Guinness with a frothy head after seventy kilometres. Maybe two. A good day in the saddle, a good day to be alive.

Boue!

The first time I see this black word on a white background on the side of the road, I have no idea what it means. The exclamation mark, though, provides the essential clue: be wary! It's a sunny morning just outside of Saint-Girons in the Midi-Pyrenees of France, only kilometres north of the Spanish border and the principality of Andorra. Early June. The *café au lait* and baguettes with marmalade we had for breakfast linger on the palate. Nine o'clock in the morning. We're cycling south and east on a quiet side road that goes to a village called Lacourt, then to the town of Oust, and finally to our destination for the day, the Col de Latrape. It's one of the climbs often featured on the Tour de France route, and that's one of the reasons we've decided on it: to test the mettle needed to go where the famous peloton has gone.

I pull up beside Kristen. We're wearing arm warmers. The *météo* on TV earlier indicated that the temperature was 12C, that it would rise to the mid twenties. Ghosts of breath puff from our lips. I ask Kristen, "What did that mean?" She shakes her head. "Dunno. Danger?" We glide along in silence. The side road we've chosen runs parallel to the Salat River, and on its far side there's a much bigger and busier carriageway, the D618. From time to time we glimpse it, and the whirr of motors and tires floats through the air when our road bends toward it.

These side roads are enjoyable. Almost always the tarmac is smooth and the lanes more than adequate for two-way traffic. Birds twitter in the bushes. Plants with bright blooms line the road, bees buzz around them. Hawks float overhead. When vehicles approach from behind, they gear down, then pass, leaving a respectful distance between themselves and our bicycles. French drivers are used to cyclists on their routes. Some toot their horns as they pass. Maybe cyclists themselves. On Sunday mornings in particular the roads are crowded with club riders, decked out in colourful jerseys, zipping from town to town in gangs of ten to fifty.

S'il vous plait, roulez doucement pour nos enfants.

This one I understand. For the sake of our children, please go slow. Sometimes the signs are accompanied by drawings by children, stick men crossing the road, children holding flowers, smiley faces. More often the signs are a prelude to the speed bumps that cross the route in most towns, slowing traffic. In Lacourt on this cool spring-like morning there are no children. But we pass an old man on an ancient bicycle with a wire basket attached to the front handlebars. He's wearing a cloth cap and has a clip on his right leg to hold his pant leg away from the chain. "*Bonjour*," we say as we pass. "*Bonjour*," he responds.

Nearly everyone in France does this. You pause on a sidewalk in a town to reconnoitre and a little old lady walking her lap dog on a leash nods at you and says, "*Messieur, Madame.*" The mustachioed delivery man looks up from the armload of baguettes he's delivering to a corner grocery and calls out, "*Allez, allez!*" Children wave crazily from the roadside. A woman hanging up laundry on a line in her yard dips her head. A reflexive grace emanates from the French countryside. Old-fashioned courtesy and good manners.

On the outskirts of Lacourt we slow for a municipal truck. Two portly workmen in green overalls are sweeping an intersection with push brooms, cigarettes dangling from their lips. They tip their heads in greeting. There's a bus shelter a little farther along. Someone has spray-painted on one of its walls: *ton terrain de jeux profitez-en, mais respite le.* It seems an odd message to be given by way of graffiti. I'm reminded of a similar graffiti I saw on a beige gymnasium wall at a private school in Canada: *Mr Hardy is a cock-sucker.* Mister? Cock-sucker? A message to a master from a deeply conflicted young man, I concluded.

The road along the Salat is lovely. Smooth surface. Almost no traffic. To one side there are rock faces where the road has been cut through; on the other the pale green and sparkling waters of the frantic Oust. At places where a gentle incline of the riverbank affords it, men with long fishing rods stand knee deep in the frothy waters. Beside them in the grass thermos bottles of coffee and brown bags are the fixings for lunch: a baguette

protrudes. Food is never far from the minds of the French. Maybe
they will catch lunch. But just in case …

Most of the ride to the town of Oust itself is on the gentle
incline. We're moving quickly, beginning to warm up by 10:00 when
we stop at the crossroads in the town and take off the arm warmers. Beside the old stone bridge at the town centre we study the
jumble of signs. One quick consult with the map and we head down
the D3 toward Seix. The grade steepens. There's a fresh breeze
blowing in our faces and for a few kilometres we take turns riding
up front to break the wind; "relaying," this is called, or "drafting."
When I pass her on one of these relays, Kristen smiles and calls
out, "Gorgeous." "Yes," I respond, "and the scenery is too." A *blague*
of long-standing that neither of us can resist.

Gravillons!

This sign is accompanied by a drawing, gravel flying up from
under the wheel of a car. Loose gravel. Though there seems to
be no more than on the verge of the previous thirty or so kilometres. We've chuckled about this before. Relative to Canadian
standards, any little defect in the road is a major event in Europe.
In Italy the government workers responsible for putting up these
signs are part of the *statale*, the state employees who are the
butt of jokes of all other Italians: they never seem to do anything,
they work a thirty-hour week, the benefits of their pension plan
are grand, they cannot be fired. Once when we saw a "bump" sign
on a road in Italy where there clearly was no bulge in the tarmac,
Kristen quipped to me, "Sergio has been out sprinkling the road
with matchsticks again."

Just past Seix we encounter a mini-peloton of cyclists wearing blue and white jerseys. They all seem to be boys, though the
man in the lead is in his forties and he wears a red helmet, where
theirs are silver and blue. We all wave. "*Bonjour, bonjour.*" The boys
make a point of looking at our machines. Theirs are good bikes,

combinations of aluminum and carbon fibre, a high-end French manufacturer. But ours garner the "Ooh-la-la" look. They're doing the descent, so they sweep past quickly. We continue climbing through densely wooded forests with waist-high grasses growing in the verges. Purple blossoms, bright yellow. The smell of ripe manure, but no barn in sight. Hidden behind the tress?

Several kilometres past Seix the D3 becomes the D81, following a tiny river, perhaps the Ustou, which twists through the countryside toward our goal. Col de Latrape is not one of the great cols. But in any Tour in which it's featured, it's an important one. Usually placed between two more demanding ascents, it's about five-and-a-half kilometres in length, covering a vertical distance of 1000 metres at an average grade of 7.5 per cent. It's demanding. The kind of climb where a rider who wishes to win a stage can "attack," with the object of leaving the peloton behind. It can be a critical moment in a given Tour. For us it will be a demanding challenge. As we approach I say to myself what I've said at the base of the cols we've attempted thus far in the Pyrenees: I'm not getting off the bike.

Chicane.

We've covered more than forty kilometres, a good warm-up for the climb ahead. At first we think we've actually started it. We pass a large sign reading "Col de Latrape: Ouvert." The grade becomes quite challenging. We gear down, expecting that around the next bend we'll begin the ascent proper. One kilometre gives way to another. Farmyards dot the valley, the tinkle of cowbells and the pungent odours of manure. It's a climb but not a col. I ask Kristen, "Are we on it yet?" I want to start the stopwatch on my cyclo-computer to see how long the climb takes us. She shakes her head. "Don't think so. Has to be steeper." Just outside of Trein de l'Ustou the grade suddenly steepens. We come round a bend in what has become a heavily forested stretch. Then we spot the sign: Col de Latrape, altitude 1100 m, 5.6 km, *moyen* 7.4%.

"Okay," Kristen calls out brightly, "see ya at the top."

But we stay together. The grade is quite demanding. In less than half a kilometre, we gear down farther, to the smallest chain ring. When the peloton of the Tour de France climbs here, thousands of fans line the route, cheering from the verges, waving flags, dousing them in cooling water. On this day, it's us and the road. Up above the sky is blue, with fluffy white clouds. Pines loom overhead. The road is two narrow lanes of tarmac, bordered by a tiny verge on each side, and precipitous drops to the receding valley below. "Aiiee," Kristen says, peering over one of the drops, "gives me the heebie-jeebies." Freefall of 1000 metres to the village rooftops below.

Sweat forms on our upper lips. Blood pounds in my temples. My heart-rate monitor reads 155, closing in on my red zone. At one of the bends there's a prospect of two green mountains in the distance, with a third snow-capped peak looming between them. "Breathtaking," Kristen says. Literally. The climb is taking my breath away.

One switchback gives way to another. Our speed drops to 12 k.p.h., and in the bends where the climbing is steepest, less than 10. We're sweating freely. The wheels of the bike rotate slowly. My heart monitor beeps a couple of times: in the red. I'm not getting off the bike, I say to myself, a point of honour that is taking its toll. We stand up for a few strokes, then go into the drops for some metres, trying to bring a variety of muscles into play. Little signs posted along the route indicate the grade of each kilometre: this one is 6.5 per cent, the last 7.5 per cent. Legs sense no difference, hearts pound on.

Zone d'amenagée.

Are there repairs ahead? We look at each other, shrug our

shoulders. The climb is difficult enough without having to manoeuvre through maintenance vehicles and workmen, orange pylons,
wheelbarrows, gravel. One bend gives way to another. No sign of
road repairs, or of road damage. So what could "amenagée" mean?

Round one bend we spot a cyclist in front of us. He's weav-
ing from side to side, clearly having a hard go of it. At the next
bend we catch up to him. A slender man in his forties, he's grunt-
ing with each breath, but as we pass he wheezes, "*Bonjour.*" We
respond and go on. At a straight stretch past the next bend,
another middle-aged man sits beside the road, his bike lying on
the grass. He's pouring water over his head, then drinking from
a plastic bottle. "*Allez, allez,*" he calls out, waving. Farther along we
pass two younger men with backpacks who also call out "*Allez*" as
we pass.

The trees thin near the summit, opening up the prospect of
the valley and the town below. Stunning. In the final kilometre the
grade drops to 4.5 per cent, the going suddenly seems easy,
and when Kristen pauses to take a photo of the switchbacks
we've just passed through, I dig down and try to open a distance
between us. But a kilometre is a long distance at a gradient, and
just at the summit she catches me. "Whatcha up to?" she asks,
wheezing and laughing. We have promised not to compete on this
trip, and for the most part we haven't.

At the summit we pull over and take photos. In a few minutes
the riders we passed below come into view and they stop and we
yak: about the climb, how far we've come today, where we're going
tomorrow. More photos. In a few minutes we'll undertake the
descent back to Seix, where we hope to have lunch. The descent
will be more demanding than the climb itself, hands clamped on
brakes, conscious on the bends of the g-forces dragging us to
the side of the road and into the precipices. At the bottom our

hands will be cramped into claws and our knees and hips will ache from clenching them through the perilous drop.

Pensez à nos enfants.

But there's café at the bottom, and lunch at a little place we noticed on the way through. Were they serving oysters? Whatever, we'll be able to try their four-course "menu" with *vin ordinaire* for ten euros each. We've earned that. The baguettes, the *cassoulet*, the cheese plate. Sometimes it comes with fresh fruit, slices of pear, plump strawberries, the juices dribble down the chin. The cook may be doing *crème brûlée*, we may be tempted by a tiny cognac with our espresso. As we glide up to the restaurant, Kristen puts out her hand for a high-five. "This is what we came to do," she says. Stole the words out of my mouth.

DEAD MAN ON A BIKE:

CRASH AND BASH

Almost from the moment we are born
little bits of us begin to fall off.
~ Gustave Flaubert

He's rolling north on Highway 26 just past St. François Xavier on the way to the bridge near Poplar Point. It's a hot summer day in late June, sun beating down on the tarmac, sweat glistening on his forearms. Soon droplets will form on his forehead and drip onto the dark glasses. The prairie is flat, the road slicing through it a grey ribbon disappearing in the shimmering distance.

Velocity: 27.5, heart rate 127. Good speed, nice pace.

He should be at the bridge in fifteen minutes. There will be shade, he will pee, he will stretch a little before the return of thirty-five kilometres. Fluffy white cloud, three crows flying high in the sky. They must be the most common creature on the face of the earth. Smart too: they've been known to drop nuts from telephone lines onto roads below in anticipation of cars coming along and breaking them open—then swoop down to pick up the fruit.

On a long ride, the mind flits. This was the road he and Bill and Brady rode down when they met Mike, cycling from the west on his jaunt across Canada; was it three summers ago? Tan and lean, Mike was wearing a plain yellow jersey and riding on hybrid tires, he looked tired when they first met up but then rejuvenated on the ride to the city and in the Ryalls' sunroom, drinking cold beer while regaling them with stories about nights in fleabag hotels and missed turnings and whatnot.

This is also the road where he ended up in the tulees after a bee got into his helmet and he banged the side of his head to shake it out—and caused himself blurred vision. Not a fall, just a brief brush with the grasses in the ditch before regaining the tarmac, the bee having flown in and then out of the helmet in the meantime: when he checked after removing it, nothing. And yet he came that close to a crash.

How many times has he crashed? The time he hit a rut on a gravel path and went straight over the bars and landed flat on his back—no damage. In England on a mountain-bike trail a drainage hole was hidden in long grass, his front wheel went into it, again over the bars and luckily not into the highway they were riding beside. He bashed into the wall at Starbucks once when he couldn't de-cleat, banged his head (helmeted) on stone. At the bottom of a hill there was a sharpish turn onto a crossing road, the tarmac was wet after rain, he skidded out and onto hip, shoulder, knee, and ankle, blew a tire, had to readjust handlebars. Two or three other times. Road rash, blood, bruises, scabs, scars.

If you ride, you fall.

You hope not to break a bone. You hope not to get hit by a car.

The wheels are whistling. This new set has flat spokes creating a high-pitched whine. A dog in a farmyard runs toward the highway: *bark bark bark.* Though big and noisy, it's no threat, they're separated by a long gravel driveway and the dog is barking to protect its territory, not to attack him. He thinks, I salute you, dog. And he laughs. He laughs because he thinks also: We're alive, dog, you and me, we're here on the planet, hearts thumping, blood coursing through veins, gritting our teeth against each other, like boxers in the ring. Bits may be falling off, as Flaubert so pointedly puts it, but we're still in the game, we're alive, dammit!

Returning from a ride to St. Adolphe, I'm pedalling at a good pace north through St. Norbert on Highway 75. St. Norbert has become a bedroom community of Winnipeg: condominiums line the highway from the strip mall that comprises the centre of the community to the overpass at the Trans-Canada Highway. In the summer months the town hosts a lively farmers' market on Saturday mornings and Wednesday afternoons.

I like this ride: ten- and twenty-minute stretches along the river in the city and out past the city limits where traffic is thin, where meadowlarks call from the fields; the pong of horse dung, the sparkle of water under the big prairie sun. There's a section in the city near Bishop Grandin Bridge where things get a bit grippy sometimes, and the kilometre of riding through St. Norbert can be dense with long-haul trucks coming into the city or making for the Trans-Canada Highway turnoff. They're usually pretty attentive to cyclists.

Suddenly on my left elbow there's a car. The driver honks his horn loudly: *blat, pay attention, I'm a car.* I ignore these vehicles; usually they're being driven by one form or another of minor cretin, trying to make a point about the importance of cars and irritation of cyclists: their point seems to be, *Get off the fuckin' road!*

This one has slowed; the driver has rolled down the window on the passenger's side. He shouts something I cannot hear and jabs one finger at the sidewalk. His face is flushed with vivid anger. I glance his way but ignore him. Best not to engage. He shouts again. I shake my head in disbelief. Drivers are not only ignorant about The Highway Traffic Act but belligerent about their ignorance. We're entitled to be out here, just as cars are: obey the traffic laws, share the road. I keep turning the pedals. *Blat.* The car remains directly at my elbow, the driver shouting incoherently but intently. This is upsetting; a lovely ride ruined by a fool. A dangerous fool. We pass the intersection at the north end of town. *Blat, blat.* I glance again at the driver: he's an older man, fat-faced, glasses, an almost bald pate. Livid cheeks. He could have a heart attack at any moment.

He could also smash into me at any moment.

He shouts again and this time I give him a dismissive wave: *bugger off.*

Just before the turn out to the highway there's a side road, Cloutier Drive; it follows the river east towards the university, and I take it, hoping to leave the car and its irate driver behind. The car follows: twenty pedal strokes, then thirty; the nose of the car is only a metre or two off my back wheel. When I speed up, it *does* too; when I slow, it slows. My chest is tight. The road ahead is deserted. What does the driver intend: hit me from behind, swing the car onto my left and then sideswipe the bike as it passes? Follow me home? Follow and continue to intimidate without doing anything else? Can I afford to wait passively in hope of the latter? Twenty pedal strokes, thirty, forty. The car is so close I can feel the heat of its engine on the backs of my legs. Ahead on my right the road opens into a construction site where a concrete driveway has been broken up preparatory to replacement. Chunks of rubble lie about. I jump up on the pedals and sprint toward it, and when I reach it, leap off the bike. My sprint has taken the driver by surprise; there's a gap of fifty metres between the car and me. I've thrown the bike aside and pick up a chunk of concrete and hurl it toward the car; it bounces on the pavement and into the ditch. The driver slows but keeps coming on; I can see he's shouting, face crimson. A second hunk of concrete bounces in front of the car and strikes its bumper; the driver lurches to a stop; begins to back up. I pause, a third piece of concrete in hand. The car moves farther back along Cloutier Drive. An SUV behind it honks its horn. The driver turns to look behind him. I hop back on the bike, pedal in terror.

Five minutes later I come out on University Crescent, having taken the ring road around the college buildings. My arms tremble, my mouth is dry, my heart hammers in the back of my throat.

Riding back from Headingley after Sunday breakfast at Nick's Inn, Kristen and I are in the shoulder alongside cycling friends we've known for some years; we call them "The Riverview Four" because they come from that neighbourhood. Paul and Eileen; Tim and Andrea. We're yakking as we pedal: Paul up front setting the pace (he still competes and likes to drive the train); Andrea just behind him because she's training for a charity ride; Eileen chatting with Kristen; Tim with me in the rear. The shoulder on this extension of Roblin Boulevard between the town of Headingley and the Perimeter Highway is wide and usually well swept: not too much rubble or gravel. (One of the things that city planners have not yet quite grasped is that building a shoulder for bicycles is only the first step in accommodating this older and more "green" form of transportation—maintaining the bike lane is equally important: too many bike lanes are unrideable because they're cluttered with litter, stones, gravel, the detritus of cars and trucks: "bagwell," named after the man who drew attention to this accumulation of debris at intersections.)

It's a pleasant enough ride. At one time, before Headingley underwent its last expansion, most of the properties along the route were farmyards, the road was little travelled by cars from the city. Birds sang in the fields, the river could be seen from the roadway, sparkling in the sun. But that recent growth has led to the issues that attend urbanization: denser car traffic, clusters of houses, and a higher volume of diesel-belching trucks. Now cyclists have to ride past Headingley to experience the quietude they used to enjoy *on the way* to Headingley. The inevitable price we pay for development.

There's a golf course about halfway along and we watch for cars coming out of its parking lot. Just past the golf course there's a wide swathe of black gravel in the shoulder: maybe a farmer has driven machinery along here. We slide over to the left, crowding the right-hand edge of the roadway. Behind us a car blats its horn—*you're in our space!* (Though technically we've not actually crossed the white line that separates shoulder from roadway.) My jaw tightens, as it always does when a horn is blatted behind me. The vehicle goes past, still honking: a black pickup. Are the most belligerent drivers on the roads inevitably behind the wheels of pickups? I'm tempted to give the finger but before I do, Tim waves at the driver, making sure he keeps his hand in the air long enough so the driver cannot miss his cheery response, fingers twiddling. Then he turns to me. "No use getting yourself in a knot about jerks," he says. "Waving takes them by surprise— *was that someone who knows me?* Even the most obnoxious jerks must experience a moment of self-doubt that could lead to better behaviour the next time." He grins. I find myself smiling as we pedal on.

With Kristen, descending Pontatoc Road in Tucson, a winding, sharp downhill from Sunrise Drive, which runs along the base of the Catalina Foothills, south to River Road. Expansive properties line the street, three-car garages, curving driveways, extensive bungalows, many with swimming pools. Cactuses of many varieties, palm trees. Blackbirds with long yellow beaks chirping from the vegetation. It's pretty in the way of desert subdivisions: brightly painted exteriors, open spaces, pervading quiet. We like this descent, Kristen especially: the grade allows the bikes to pick up speed with every kilometre, the sweeping curves add the degree of excitement that comes when the road ahead is momentarily blocked from view, then opens suddenly into the next curve—or series of curves. The heart surges with the sudden, sharp, and short plunges that characterize these drops off the foothills. There are very few cars; many cyclists pedal up and down: nods of the head, waves, cheery greetings.

We come to the bottom. Behind us a car is honking, *blat blat*, as we make the right turn onto River Road. *Blat, blat.* Have we taken the right-hander too wide, crossed the white line into the vehicle lane? It cannot be; the bike lane here, as in most places in Tucson, is wide. The car comes up beside us, a black convertible, the white-haired man inside holding up a badge and pointing right, directing us to pull over. We slow. I call to Kristen: "What's this?" She shakes her head as she comes up alongside. The old guy has put the nose of his car across the bike lane, so we have no choice but to pull up.

"You can't ride there," he screams at us, still flashing his badge. His flushed face suddenly reminds me of photos of Franco, screaming from a podium.

I shout back: "What? We—"

"Damn you cyclists, all over the damn road. You can't—"

"We were in the bike lane. We still are."

"I should write you up."

"For what?"

"You're all over the road. You always are, you damn bikers."

"You're out of your mind, you old bugger."

Kristen has moved her bike closer to mine. "Wayne, Wayne," she says, "Let me handle this."

"What do you mean? This old asshole—"

"I should damn well report you."

Kristen puts one hand on my shoulder. "On what authority? I should report you for impersonating a policeman."

The old guy's face goes livid. He puts the badge he's been waving down and out of sight. Cars behind us have slowed. A few horns toot.

"That's right," I shout. "Piss off. Just piss off out of here."

"Wayne, calm down, Wayne. He's going, he's going now."

The old guy's car jerks back suddenly, as he reverses into the vehicle lane, then screeches away. Behind and beside him, car horns are honking. He swerves into the bike lane ahead, nearly hitting the curb, then rights the car and roars away.

I turn to Kristen. "What was that?" I can hardly get the words out.

"No idea. Frustrated rent-a-cop, security guard?"

"That badge was not a cop's badge."

"No."

"He had no right." We both swig from our water bottles. We start to pedal again. There's a Starbucks ahead where we often stop for coffee. It will be a good place to gear down—in both senses.

"Road Nazi."

"Got that right."

"Road Nazis," Kristen repeats with a long sigh.

Doing the El Tour charity ride around Tucson in mid November. Ten thousand participants. The year previous I finished first in the old farts' division, sixty and older, and Kristen finished fourteenth among all women doing the distance we chose that time: 45 miles, 75 kilometres.

We're to the north of the city and moving west, making the long crescent that swings south, eventually, and back to the heart of the metropolis. Beneath us the road is somewhat lumpy, but the riding is at a brisk pace. Most of the riders doing the El Tour strictly to raise money for hospital research have been dropped; the pack is now made up of focused cyclists, recreational riders, true, but focused nonetheless.

El Tour is fun. Traffic is controlled, no worries about road rage. You meet a lot of people from Tucson and many other places: California, Colorado, Australia, other Canadians. You ride along with a group for a while, and then it breaks up; a couple on a tandem goes past; you hitch onto their back wheel, and then another group forms, new people to chat with, though most of the time you're working hard.

We move up beside a guy wearing the full Livestrong kit: bib shorts, bright yellow jersey, helmet. He's in his forties, maybe, stocky and well-tanned. "You're all decked up," I say pleasantly, nodding at his clothing. "My mom bought it for me," he says, grinning. I nod. "You a cancer survivor?" He shakes his head. "No, nothing like that. My mom just wanted me to have it." We ride on. Ahead there's a climb coming; Kristen has gone a bit up the road. He says, "You're wearing the yellow band." I glance down at it. It's been on my wrist for about five years; I've never taken it off; I often forget it's there. I hesitate, glance at him, then take the plunge. "I'm no fan of Lance Armstrong," I begin, "but I'm living with a terminal cancer." I can never be sure which of these two remarks might spark an unhappy response. He looks at me quizzically, making sure he's understood correctly. My gaze tells him he has. "Hey, guys," he calls out. The three riders ahead are apparently his pals, they swivel their heads and slow their pedalling. "This guy's got cancer," he calls out. "Shit, no kidding," one says. They all slow, absorbing the Livestrong guy and me among them. "Jesus," says another. The third guy nods and purses his lips, gives me the thumbs up, but does not say anything. He doesn't need to. I've noted the way he's nodded, and he's seen that I've seen. I swallow back the lump in my throat. We pedal on toward the climb ahead.

Riding back from Assiniboine Park on a July afternoon, I'm on the Proflex and following a footpath that goes across a grassy knoll at the railway yards at Jubilee. This is a nice section of a ride that takes me north from where we live into the park, where the roads are quiet: ducks paddle in the duck pond, the scent of animals wafts from behind Frost fences. In front of me a guy in a blue jacket with shoulder patches stands on the track. As I approach, he waves his arms at me. I slow, then stop.

"Get off your bike," he commands.

I stay where I am, straddling the top tube.

"Off," he blurts.

"You're kidding." I see that his patches have CN stencilled on them in red.

"You're on CN property," he says, "you're trespassing."

"I've ridden this path a hundred times. So do thousands of others. Look how it's worn."

He glances down, but when he looks up, his mouth has hardened. "No more you don't, you smart-aleck bike riders."

"Christ almighty,"

"I need ID," he blurts. "Show me ID. I'm going to write you up. A citation."

I snort. "A citation."

"You're on private property."

"I don't carry any," I say. "And I don't think you have the authority to ask."

"Authority, eh? You don't, eh?" He's middle-aged, maybe fifty, greying at the temples, pot-belly, fat face, blocky torso.

"Christ," I say, "we ride here all the time. And there's no posting."

"Right back there."

I look over my shoulder. There's a tin rectangle attached to a metal stake. I recall seeing it before; recently maybe. PRIVATE PROPERTY. "It says nothing about trespassing."

"Doesn't hafta."

"So you say."

"So I do."

If my face is as red as his, we're both standing at the open door of an angry furnace. I start to turn my bike around.

"You're not going nowhere," he growls. He's reached his hand out, as if to grab my arm. My hands are trembling. This guy is spoiling for a scrap, he's got a look in his eye I know well. Bully.

"I wouldn't do that," I say. "That's got assault written all over it."

"You think so?"

"I think you want to give people a warning. Rather than start threatening them with arrest and whatnot. People who've been using a footpath for years without being hassled." I glare into his grey eyes. My heart is thumping, my mouth dry. I'm wondering, Could this actually come to blows, me and this fifty-year-old bully trading punches on the CN grassy knoll?

"I should write you up," he says. I know from his tone that he will not, that I've won out. Though he's won too. I'll have to turn around and find another route home. "Jesus," I mutter.

"I'm just doing my job," he asserts.

"That's what Adolph Eichmann said."

"Hey," he shouts. "You—"

"Forget it."

I clip into the bike's pedals and begin to move off.

"You're lucky," he shouts, voice cracking. "I wrote a smartass cyclist like you up yesterday. I should have wrote you up."

Once the bike is rolling, I mutter back at him, "I'm surprised, I'm surprised you know how to put pen to paper."

Pedalling north from Cahors, a college town in the Dordogne region of southern France. A hot day in mid August, but a glorious one. Blue skies above, hawks riding air currents, the chirring of insects in the ditches. The road is quiet, as are most roads in rural France: winding lanes with short, sharp climbs into hilltop towns, fields of vines on both shoulders. The area is known for a very dark, aromatic red wine made from the Malbec grape, the "black wine of Cahors."

Up ahead are two famous chateaux, for which the region is also known, *bastides* built during the Hundred Years War. Castles, actually, perched on hilltops, from which invading armies could be spotted, the reasons the castles exist.

Kristen is having a bad day. She woke with an irritated stomach, did not eat breakfast, stayed in the hotel room while I went out for *café au lait*. Her face is red, she keeps falling behind. Our pace drops to 15 k.p.h. Sweat beads her forehead and chin. "Still?" I ask.

"My gut, yeah. I got food poisoning last night."

"We ate the same thing. That dog at the next table, too."

"I had the pâté."

"Ah, the pâté."

We pedal on, moving slower. We've made reservations at a hotel about eighty kilometres down the road. We've gone thirty or so, fifty remain. Up and down hills in the heat. She's not going to make it. I think this, but neither of us says anything.

Five kilometres, eight. We enter a village. Noon has come and gone. It's one o'clock and shops are closing up, proprietors heading home for lunch. In villages in rural France the bakery closes at noon, the deli at one, though the restaurants remain open until two.

In the centre of the village we pull over. "I need water," Kristen says. She's been glugging from her bottle all morning. I prop my bike against a lamppost. The shop we're in front of is a bakery, the proprietor just pulling down the metal shutter over the window. "*Un moment*," I call out. Just then I hear a gurgling sound come from Kristen behind me. I look back. She's bent over the gutter, vomiting. I rush across the sidewalk. The shop's shutter is down and the proprietor has gone inside, but the door remains open. I rush inside. "*Ma femme*," I say, motioning back behind me, "*ma femme …*" A woman has come forward through a curtain at the rear of the shop. "*Fermé, monsieur*," she says, "close."

"*Ma femme*," I insist, "*ma femme a mal à la gorge.*"

Behind me Kristen wheezes out, "*Estomac*." She's propped against the doorway, partly bent over. "*Mal à l'estomac.*"

"*Ah, madame*," the woman says. She rushes forward. "*Pauvre madame.*"

Kristen's face is a pallid rictus. She holds one hand over her belly.

The woman shouts to her husband, who emerges in a moment with a bottle of cold water. Which Kristen drinks. I thank him, thank them both. I say, "We ride to Touzac. I don't think my wife can make it. Is there a taxi we can hire?"

"*Ah, oui*," the woman begins, "*le taxi*—"

"Taxi, humph," the man says. "I drive. I drive madame."

Despite our protests that he will miss his lunch, the man

waves his arms, stomps out to a car out front, puts Kristen's bike in the trunk, and helps her into a seat. I say again, "Hotel le Source Bleu, Touzac."

"*Mais oui,*" he says, "Touzac."

I push a fifty-euro note toward him.

"*Messieur,*" he says, "*mais non, c'est ici Luzech, ce n'est pas Paris.*"

I turn to his wife. She raises both hands: nothing to do with me.

I lean in on Kristen's side. "I'll be maybe two hours. Take care."

"You too. And don't forget to eat lunch."

The car roars off in a cloud of blue smoke. It's at that moment that I think, I've just put my sick wife into a car with a man whose name I do not know and he's roared off with her into the French countryside. *Ce n'est pas Paris.*

DEAD MAN ON A BIKE:

COUNTING PEDAL STROKES

The bicycle is just as good company as most husbands,
and when it gets old and shabby a woman can get a new one
without shocking the entire community.
~ Ann Strong

Mid-morning on a sunny but chilly day in Wisconsin. They've ridden for almost an hour along a valley and have come to the foot of a climb onto a ridge. They're on county U, which climbs to a highway up on the ridge, #88, a busy road between large rural towns that also leads to county N, a ridge ride.

The climb starts fast, as they often do in this area, the first half kilometre or so the steepest. They have no idea how long the ascent is—or how steep. Most in the area are no longer than four kilometres, though a few are quite demanding: 10 per cent. And once, near Pine Creek, there was a section at 18 per cent. At the top they were going so slow DMB nearly fell off the bike.

This is a good one: he gears down once in the opening half kilometre and then again within a few hundred metres. One gear left. He likes to keep the "granny gear" in reserve, a fallback in case the ascent steepens suddenly. There are a lot of switchbacks. On the sixth or seventh they hear an engine changing gears above them. And in a few moments a pickup comes around the bend in front of them, loaded with hay bales. When it passes, the guy driving lifts one finger off the wheel. DMB nods back. Straw swirls around them as the pickup goes past.

Kristen sneezes.

He's sweating, feels the climb in the quads, begins to count pedal strokes. Fifty sitting, then thirty standing, bringing different muscles into play. Feels good. Then eighty sitting, fifty standing. Alternating between positions takes considerable energy but relieves the back and hip muscles. And the counting gives the illusion of accomplishing something.

At an opening in the woods, they look down on the valley they've just come from: a farm house, barn, silos, cattle in the meadows. The babble of running water, crickets chirring, the scrunching of wheels moving slowly over rough tarmac. Is this the fifth or sixth such climb they've done on this trip? The first one was difficult; around Winnipeg there are no hills; but each successive climb has been easier; the legs are toughening in.

He's moving at a good pace but not pushing things. Kristen could climb this much quicker. Which used to bother him, the old macho thing asserting itself; but those days are past. DMB is in his sixties; he's got a terminal cancer; he's lucky to be out on a bike at all. Much less riding up to a hundred kilometres a day and climbing up ridge roads. "Go ahead," he says to her, "see how far it is to the top."

She dances off and in a few moments disappears around the next bend. He's still counting strokes. Fifty sitting, fifty standing. Bees and wasps buzz about; on the road butterflies sit and fold wings in and out. Two days ago a fox came out of a cornfield onto the road ahead of them, studied them quizzically a moment or so, then darted back into the cornstalks. It's deer country; they've seen a number. Skunks, a badger, what appeared to be bear poop on the roadside. Wonderfully backwoodsy.

Kristen comes back down the road. "About five hundred metres to the top," she says as she passes. In a few moments he can hear her panting behind him, having turned in the road below him before catching up again.

It's flatter toward the top and the pedalling becomes easier: cadence jumps from the low 60s to the 70s. Okay, he's reached the crest. Though his heart rate never exceeded 140, the climb was taxing in other ways. But now comes the ride on the ridge, rolling between fields for ten kilometres or so at a breezy 25 or 30 k.p.h. All good, all clear ahead.

More and more come the days—and nights—when a malaise settles over my whole being, like the stuffy-headedness of a cold, a thickness of the spirit that erodes the will to go on. Fighting cancer over a long period of time is not easy. It wears you down physically, tiring you out; it blackens your mind and leads you to the precipice and the abyss. Oh, what the hell, why go on, why put up with the thickness in the throat, the pains near the liver, the puffing at the top of the staircase; listlessness as the sun sinks in the west, marking the end of another day?

I'm sick as often as I'm healthy, and the dark clouds of depression thicken on the horizon of my spirit often. Cancer is getting the better of me. On the worst days I wonder how many more days the Fates have apportioned me: less than a thousand? more?

Three years, maybe five. No, not so many as five. Such thoughts force me into denial, to blocking out median survival rates and calculations about mortality from the jumble of thoughts racing this way and that inside my skull: will I see Andrew graduate with his engineering degree?

I lie in bed at 3:00 in the night, curled into the foetal position and staring out the window: there's pain and there's discomfort. But more important, there are dark thoughts that end with closing the eyes and thinking maybe the struggle has gone on long enough, maybe it's time to accept defeat. Why do we go on, anyway? Trudge through dreary days when the grey in the sky is matched by the grey in the heart? That kind of thinking can go on for some time. But then a little voice says: *oh, stop feeling sorry for yourself; get on with it, be a man.* So I draw in a few deep breaths and say, all right, all right, we'll forge on.

Willed obliviousness, then. Forging on in the face of facts.

The sickness descends on my days. I lose the desire to do things. I lie on the couch under a blanket and watch TV. I drop into long naps and wake with aching guts and a murky brain. Hours pass. It was 1:30 when I lay down on the sofa; now it's coming on for 5:00. I meant to call a friend and set up a lunch date; that will have to wait. Soon Kristen and Andrew will be home for supper.

I'm the cook in our house, and I like it, but there are evenings when I push away the blanket with great reluctance and cross into the kitchen to prepare our evening meal on leaden legs. Go through the motions over the stove. I bring the plates to the table and the dish I've prepared revolts me. It's a simple pasta dish, easy to digest on days when the gut is roiling and boiling. I come to the table and sit with Andrew and Kristen and the food brings bile to the back of my throat, I want to vomit. But I do not push the plate away. It's important to eat. I have to keep up my strength. This is an old saw of my mother's from childhood days when we were ill with colds and flus: "you have to eat something, you have to keep up your strength." Almost sixty years later she's there inside me still: waggling her index finger. So I push back a forkful. I can tell it's tasty, a savoury combination of garlic, olive oil, pepperoncini, chopped parsley with a spaghettini, topped by freshly ground parmesan. But I have to choke it back. One forkful, two. We chat about this and that. Kristen has poured a glass of wine for each of us, a passable Malbec from the Cahors region of France, but in my mouth it's vinegar. I take a sip, push the glass away. My head is falling forward as I choke back another forkful of pasta—and then another: six, eight, ten. The food wants to come back up my esophagus. I swallow it down. I listen to the conversation and forge on.

I like the pun in "forge." On the surface the word suggests that we do things despite how difficult or trying they might be. It's a concept I'm fond of, along with *endurance* and *commitment*. It's a word about determination, about willpower. But the secondary meaning of "forge" is with me always, too: I'm fabricating, putting up a front, passing something off as something it is not. At the table with Kristen and Andrew I try to appear strong, masterful. I'm doing fine. I nod. They know better, but they go along. We're all involved in a little conspiracy inside the house: Dad's putting up the good fight, he's okay. Outside of the house, it's much the same: I meet friends for breakfast, or coffee, or lunch, and I put up the brave front: I'm fine, I'm doing okay. My friends nod and smile, but I can tell from the way their eyes shift from mine to the cup in front of them that they're not so sure. Often we do talk for a few minutes about the actual state of things inside my unravelling body. I have good friends; they care; they're prepared to listen. But my cancer battle has been going on for twenty years. We're all tired of it. I'm tired of being a cancer patient; they're tired of dealing with a cancer patient. I sometimes wonder if some of them haven't reached their limit and cannot help thinking: *oh, just die already!* We can only endure so much of someone else's suffering or grief. A kind of self-preservation instinct kicks in: be done with it already, let me get on with things. I don't blame anyone who feels this. I'd most likely feel it myself, if I were in their shoes.

But we smile, we chat amicably about this and that—their careers, children, the state of the world. We forge on. Like the eating, we know it's important to keep up strength. To hold up the chin. Both require a certain degree of willed stupidity in the face of the reality.

Something similar happens with the bike. I once was a good rider and took great pleasure from long or challenging rides. I can do very little of either any longer. An outing of fifty kilometres is now as tiring as a ride of a hundred used to be. Climbing a mountain takes tremendous determination: I will have a sore back the next day; I may provoke a sciatic nerve flare-up; the strained hamstring I live with permanently now will be worse for a couple of days; I'll be exhausted. Despite knowing this, I put on the latex, clip into the pedals, hop onto the saddle. I go out there. Riding the bike is not so much pleasure any more. Often it's quite the opposite. I don't really want to go out there and turn the pedals, but I have to go. I go out there because it's good for me: riding the bike maintains muscle tone, it takes me out of myself for several hours, it puts the heart to the test. It may even provoke the desire to eat a big meal at the close of the day.

Deep breath, then. Forge on.

So. What sustains me is the bike. It's comforting to go out there, hear the wheels whirring below, feel the muscles in the legs, in the back straining with effort, straining with life force. The sun shines down, the wind teases the face, the little critters hop and scuttle along the side of the road, intent on their little critter lives. Heartbeat jumps from 80 beats per minute to 110 and then wavers up and down between 120 and 130. The heart beats blood, the mind is alert to the dangers of the road, eyes scan the tarmac, ears listen for the sounds of car tires behind. I'm alive, I'm on the bike, I'm vital.

It need not be a bike. There's a woman I know in Calgary who's fought the C for a number of years now, really fought. Given just months, she's thrown herself into life, *at* life with a manic passion that has won the hearts of thousands of people and astounded her doctors. She's taken an unusual tack: she dresses up in wild costumes, pastiches of Egyptian princesses, heroines from movies like *Avatar*, fusions of the classic and contemporary. Her hairstyles are eye-opening swirl-ups and concoctions from speculative cinema. Though given a death sentence, she has defied it, travelled to cities to see theatric performances and art exhibitions. An exhibition herself, in her stunning getups, makeup, hair stylings, she draws people's eyes and she greets them with bright smiles and mock boogies. She refuses to give in; she declines to give up. She dazzles. And there's not a bicycle in sight.

Her life is a performance. And a statement: I am here, I defy the odds. I live.

DEAD MAN ON A BIKE:

GET THEE BEHIND ME, SATAN

Never a bad day to ride.

A chilly day in October, 4C when they went out earlier for the coffee ride to Starbucks. Not much warmer now, maybe 7C. And a north wind. Brrr. DMB is wearing a skullcap and over that, a toque. Wind-resistant jacket, tights.

Why is he out here?

It's the exercise: working the legs, taxing the lungs, keeping fit. That's one explanation. Play a little tennis, go out for hockey, ride the bike, throw weights, get on the wind-trainer on days when nothing else is possible.

Then, too, once you start exercising, it's like most other things, the routine of doing it takes over; that's the kind of creatures humans are. We're animals. We live by routine. Deer go down to the watering hole on the same track every time, setting themselves up for easy ambush by predators. Routine. Maybe that's it.

Or how about this: in a recent book he's confessed to being obsessive about riding his road bike. Obsession. He knows a thing or two about that.

And who is DMB fooling? Without realizing it, riding the bike has become something of an obsession with him, a way of proving to himself that he is not succumbing to cancer, a way of saying to the disease: "Get thee behind me, Satan."

On this blustery, cool, and cloudy morning he arrives at Crescent Park, only a few kilometres from home. You can make a loop around the park of just over two kilometres; and there's a long flat stretch running along the river. So it's a training ride, warming up for the twenty minutes it takes to get the park, ditto on the return, and thirty-five minutes of something a bit more demanding: today wind sprints. The book he has, Chris Carmichael's *Lance Armstrong's Training Program,* calls for sprints of thirty seconds all-out followed by a minute and a half of recovery, then another sprint, five sprints in total. He tweaks that for his own situation: sprints for fifty seconds, then recovers for the time it takes to come back to the place on the loop where he jumps up to begin; recovery of about three-and-a-half minutes. Six sprints.

The first one is the hardest, jumping up and hammering. And

keeping it going at top output for the fifty seconds. When he sits, he checks the heart-rate monitor: 160.

After the sprint, you carry speed into the recovery part of the ride.

He passes an older couple walking hand-in-hand toward him. Why does that always make his chest expand? Then a guy walking his dog. DMB eyes the dog until he's past: you never know what "barker" is going to do—jump at you, try to bite your leg? He likes dogs, but bicycles and dogs don't mix well. Here's two women "power-walking," humping along, arms swinging violently. Marching to Pretoria.

Sprint two: heart rate jumps to the mid 160s. The second and third sprints feel the best, sometimes even the fourth: heart rate up, legs into it. By the fifth he begins to tire, and the heart rate is now quite high. The end of the sixth is welcome. He checks the computer as he goes into rest mode: max speed: 46.3; average heart rate: 147; max heart rate: 169. He was working.

Okay, then, once more around the park in coast mode. Here's a woman walking three dogs, their leashes becoming entangled. And a guy jogging, wearing shorts and a T-shirt. WTF! It's cold out here, man. It doesn't seem to bother some people. A dead squirrel, smushed by a car. Tough luck, little buddy. But why did you have to cross the road? Why does anyone have to cross the road?

DMB is warm now. When he's doing warm-down stretches at home, the muscles will feel pliable. Nice. *Get thee behind me, Satan!*

Bordeaux, from "bord" and "d'eau," meaning beside the water. One of France's most important sea ports, situated at the mouth of the Gironde River and flanked by the Médoc to the north and west, the wine areas of the Libourne to the east, with Toulouse to the south and Nantes to the north on the eastern side of the Gironde. Famous for its wines. But we've come to cycle.

We manoeuvre through the town we're staying in,

Saint-Laurent, and in moments cross the secondary highway traversing the Médoc north and south and we're on a quiet tertiary highway heading east into the famous wine regions. Saint-Julien and Beychevelle are quaint towns, smaller than Saint-Laurent, where dogs wander along the sidewalk, children ride bikes, and locals amble across the road in front of us as we breeze through. We pass Château Gloria, a famous but modest place, and then the magnificent Château Beychevelle where the D101 gives way to the D2, which runs through the wine country north and south. We turn north toward Paulliac and pass beautiful châteaux situated on the rises in the undulating terrain. These once were "castles," and their location on the hilltops made them difficult in the medieval times to assail. This road is busier than the D101, but still comfortable riding. The tarmac is good, the rolling grades pleasant to ascend and descend. Cars whiz past, but the drivers are courteous and leave plenty of space between their vehicles and us. Occasionally someone honks and waves, a cyclist presumably. It's late May and the plants along the roadside are in bloom, their bright reds and yellows eye-catching and their thin fragrance pleasant to the nostrils.

It's a delightful morning, the temperature in the high teens with the prediction of mid twenties to come. Overhead the sun beats down, but there's a cooling breeze and the occasional cloud in the blue sky. The smells of turned earth, the smells of the terroir of the Bordeaux region.

Though the terrain is rural and the fields stretch as far as the eye can see, there are no sheep dotting the hillsides, no cattle with tinkling bells, no farming on these hectares. Every field is a vineyard, whether on the slopes or on the flats, some gigantic, perhaps as much as two kilometres square, others not so big. Rows of staked vines. On these vineyards a few people work, moving slowly down the rows, bending at each vine. We're moving so fast on our bicycles it's difficult at first to see what they're doing—checking for bugs, clipping bits off the plants, spraying? Whatever they're doing, it's exacting work and slow, the rows stretch by the dozen across the fields and each one tapers into a needle at its far reach.

We move along briskly. North of Beychevelle the highway undulates and the rhythms of cycling up and down hills occupy us as the châteaux slip past on both sides, the Gironde in the distance to our right, the east. It takes very little time to reach Pauillac and the famous Château Mouton Rothschild, a massive building situated among hectares of vines. Tourist buses and cars crowd the parking lot: signs indicate that tours provide a look at the wine-making process and samplings of the famous vintages (at exorbitant prices).

The D2 north of Pauillac on the way to Saint-Estèphe is charming. For kilometres tall trees, willows of some kind, flank both sides of the roadway, forming an arch. We spot a nuclear plant on the far shore of the Gironde, and then a tall three-masted ship, reminiscent of the *Bluenose*, impressively sailing down the river from the north, its white sails and amber masts winking in the sunshine. The road past Saint-Estèphe is a little rougher than previously, pebbly tarmac. *Gravillons*, the signs read, and show gravel spraying up from a car tire. Road signs dot the route: *Pensez à Nos Enfants, Route Inondable*. Along one stretch there are tall trees with foliage only near the tops, like palms, and in one of these cranes have built a nest, a huge circular affair that is eye-catching and magnificent.

The cathedral at Saint-Estèphe is small by the standards of the great ones, but arresting. It's situated in the old town square, which is a cobblestone courtyard. The stone steps of the church have been worn into concave dishes by centuries of shuffling feet, the wooden door latch is scarred by fingernails and worn a dark brown, almost black. Inside the grey stone floor gives off a musty pong reminiscent of moss and stagnant water. The transept has stained glass windows depicting the trials of Jesus. Our shoes echo in the high lofts of the ceiling. We study the glass windows and in a side chapel near the entrance I put coins in the box and light a candle for my father, gone now more than a decade. We tiptoe out as a white-haired lady comes in with a tiny brown dog on a red leash.

Outside we pause in the square and watch a flock of pigeons poking about near a trash bin. They really are spectacularly stupid creatures, sitting for hours on high wires, cooing, crapping, bobbing their heads as if they're having trouble swallowing, pecking in the gravel. They always seem to be hungry and they never seem to actually eat anything.

We step into the *maison de vin*, across the square from the church. They have racks of recent vintages from the region. The wines are attractively displayed. We look at a Château Le Boscq, which we have at home. It sells here for thirty euros, about what we pay back home. Air transport has made foreign and exotic items readily available in all corners of the world, but it has also meant the levelling of prices from one place to another. It used to be that leather goods in Italy, and wine and cheese in France, were inexpensive compared to the costs at home. But now all that has changed. Maybe our world, called by many the *global village*, should be called the *level village*.

On the bicycles past Saint-Estèphe we settle into a rhythm, drafting each other for two minutes at a time into the headwind from the north, which feels to be about 30 k.p.h. Little settlements flit by. The farther north in the "bas Médoc," the more cattle there are in the fields, the fewer giant vineyards with their impressive châteaux. This is the country of Cru Bourgeois and Domaine wines, some as tasty in their way as the famous vintages, and at a fraction of the cost. Vehicular traffic thins. Hawks drift overhead. On the warm tarmac at Port de Goulee two mallards sun themselves and we stop and take a snapshot of them before a lorry approaches and startles them into flight, the greens and reds of the drake suddenly vivid against the blue sky. It's lunch time as we approach Verdon at the northernmost tip of the Médoc. We pull up to an establishment with a menu-board outside, indicating that the lunch on offer is soup, choice of a *confit* or *cassoulet*, and dessert. A bottle of *vin de table* comes with the meal, all at the modest price of ten euros per person. The place is filled with locals, workmen in overalls, families with children, businessmen in suits, retired couples, all busy at con-versation and consumption.

We're greeted by the clatter of cutlery and the florid-faced woman in charge, who points us to a table. In a moment a waitress comes to our table. She is tall and slender and resembles Olive Oyl from the Popeye comic strip, short hair, a neck like a goose. "The *confit d'oie*," she adds, "*c'est superbe*." She's recommending the goose, and she pats the nape of her neck while she waits for us to decide. Kristen and I look at each other and can barely suppress our snickers. We order one *cassoulet* and one *confit* of goose.

Both turn out to be delicious.

There's always a trick to be acquired in travel, and one in France is to locate these modest eating places, habituated by the locals. "Menu restaurants," we call them, after the black chalk menus posted outside their doors, indicating the fare on offer and its price per person. The food is hearty, if not spectacular, the service friendly and quick, the atmosphere bright and buoy-ant. And for the equivalent of thirty-five dollars two cyclists can enjoy a filling and satisfying meal, a litre of *vin ordinaire* included.

A ferry connects Verdon to the largish port town of Royan on the eastern side of the river, and the trip takes only thirty minutes, so we're on the bikes heading south on the D25 shortly after noon. The views from the highway on this side of the Gironde are fetching but the road is busy for the first thirty or so kilometres. At the little town of Montagne the highway becomes the D145, a smaller and much less travelled route, though the views of the Gironde on our right are as charming. There are hills on this side of the Gironde, some quite demanding, and the going is challenging but not off-putting, taxing climbs of several kilometres followed by breezy descents that cool the arms and legs, which are absorbing serious UV rays in the midday sun. At the low spots between climbs we chat briefly. "This is what we came to do," Kristen says. "Great ride," we agree, and prepare for the next ascent.

At the apex of one of these, just past La Rive, we spot a roadside kiosk advertising Vente de Pineau. We've noticed a number of signs featuring Pineau and we pull up at the kiosk to find out what it is: a beverage, we assume, from the bottles depicted on the roadside advertisements. An elderly man wearing spectacles and a short-sleeved checkered shirt stands on the other side of the counter. Pineau, he informs us, is an aperitif, made of the grapes growing on the vines behind the kiosk, a fortified wine that is a specialty of the region, Charentes, he tells us, as Cognac is of the Cognac region to the east. It comes in white and red varieties, he explains, as he pours us one of each in sherry-style glasses. It's dense and sweet and lovely, and if we weren't on bicycles, we tell him, we'd take a bottle. But alas. He laughs. "C'est bon," he says, and asks us where we're from and how we're enjoying our stay in France. "C'est bon," we tell him.

The road plunges almost immediately and then climbs steeply into Saint-Thomas, where we spot a sign, "Sport-Café Bar." We pull the bicycles over and step inside. The place is empty at 2:30, but the proprietor is behind the bar. "Bonjour," he says, and immediately it's obvious from his accent that he's English. He's from Manchester, it turns out, and he and his wife have been running the bar for less than a year, but happily and successfully, it turns out, as he tells us his story while we wait for a large plate of frites we've ordered to accompany our glasses of beer. "Oh, my head," he says, "I've got the hangover today." He laughs and adds, "Big party last night." He pours three large glasses of water, one for himself, which he downs in one go. The French, he says, do not easily welcome newcomers to their village, but they like the bar and they've grown to like him. A former baggage handler, he enjoys being a small businessman. Government red tape can be an issue, but he's learning how to deal with it—or rather, his wife, Toni, is: he works in the bar and she does the "business end." They bought the place on a whim, attached living quarters included, and they're making a go of it. "Imagine," he says, "a bloke from Manchester who couldn't speak a word of French when I came over, making a living in this little town, with my kids growing up fluent in the lingo."

The morning breezes that struck our faces as we headed north have freshened and are now at our backs as we cycle south toward the town of Blaye and the ferry that crosses the Gironde in the south. A few cows stand in the fields on the flats near the Gironde. The views of the river and the terrain sloping towards it are lovely, especially at the crests of the hills, where the eye can view the landscape of both shorelines as well as the river in the middle ground. The vineyards run down the slopes and onto the flats. Bright orange and red poppies grow in the ditches. Crows flap overhead and caw. The sweet odour of manure is on the air. The tires of the bicycles whirr along. We're conscious that we must make it to Blaye to catch the final ferry of the day at 6:00. At Saint-Ciers the D146 becomes the D255, and somewhat busier as the vehicles whiz by at the end of the workday. The terrain, which undulated and challenged the legs from Royan to

Saint-Ciers, is flat and the road mostly straight, running through marshland, with canal-like channels on both sides. Cranes feed in the waters and flap up heavily and fly off. Signs warn: ROUTE INONDABLE. A farmer on a field cuts hay with a tractor-drawn implement. A donkey is tied to a stake in a field and it brays at us as we pass. It's a pretty ride, despite the thickening traffic near Blaye, a busy, commercial town with expensive shops and a number of attractive hotels along its riverfront.

The ferry ride to Lamarque takes about forty minutes. Standing up front we enjoy the spray and the breezes off the river. Couples stand at the ferry railing and chatter. Take snapshots of the town as the ferry docks. Our cheeks are hot, and our legs are a bit stiff as we remount for the final section of the ride, from Lamarque back to Saint-Laurent. A long day in the saddle is coming to a close. We're tired and hungry, sweaty and depleted. Showers await, cold beer from the bar at our hotel. But it's north again on the D2 heading to Beychevelle. Lovely tiny purple and white flowers grow in the ditches. The road curves and undulates. On the straight stretches we put our heads down and freewheel along as briskly as we can. Tractors are coming off the vineyards, too, spidery things whose cabs sit up high to avoid damaging the vines, and with movable arms that resemble tentacles, mechanical arms which are employed in spraying the vines. They look like giant robotic insects. Kristen calls them "spraying mantis."

It's been a long ride, some 140 kilometres in a hot sun, and back at our modest *auberge* we're happy to drink a couple cold beer and remove the clinging latex cycling gear. Stretch and stretch out. Supper, too, is welcome. The locals at the bar nod at us and say "bonsoir." When we answer back, they realize we speak French and a woman in her fifties says, "*Vous allez par vélo, non?*" We say yes, we travel by bicycle. "*Où?*" she asks, where? And we sketch in briefly our ride for the day. A gap-toothed man listening in says,

"That far on a bicycle? I get tired going that far in my car." They all laugh. The woman explains that she's a retired schoolteacher and travels around France herself. "Have you visited the cathedral in Saint-Estèphe?" she asks. "*Très belle.*" We tell her yes, and she nods her approval. "*Très belle,*" she repeats. "Not so grand as some, but very pretty. We are very proud of it. You must visit too the sand dunes at Lacanau. Biggest sand dunes in France." One of the men adds, "In all of Europe." The others nod their agreement. We tell them that's on our itinerary for tomorrow. The gap-toothed man says, "It's sixty kilometres each way. You're doing that *par vélo?*" We nod. He shakes his head and says something to the others, which we don't quite catch, and they all laugh. Crazy tourists. It's good-humoured fun at our expense, more bemused admiration than anything else, and in a moment they raise their glasses to us. "*Vive le vélo,*" they say. We raise ours in return: "*Vive la France.*"

We have an espresso each and say "bonsoir." Take a brief stroll around town before the welcoming, cool sheets of bed.

DEAD MAN ON ABIKE:

TOPPING THE ICON

Cycling is a constant lesson in humility.
~ Louison Bobet, three-time winner of Le Tour de France

The sign on the bend up ahead on a steel post at about the eight-foot level reads: "6." The Alps, France. DMB is climbing the famous Alpe d'Huez, with its striking twenty-one switchbacks. Late August, 2013.

The Alpe d'Huez has, in cycling terms, reached the status of iconic. It is not the most difficult climb in France. It is not even the most difficult climb in the Alps. But it has garnered mythic status. So, if you go cycling in the Alps, you must climb the Alpe d'Huez: 13.2 kilometres at an average grade of 8.1 per cent and a maximum of 14 per cent. And all those *virages*, each numbered from bottom to top.

Up ahead of DMB is Kristen, spinning along nicely. DMB is grinding it out: ten kilometres per hour drops to nine coming out of *virage* #6 and then drops to seven. Much slower and the bike will begin to wobble. He keeps the pedals turning. Heart rate 150 becomes 154. Soon it will hit 156, the beginning of his red zone.

As the road straightens past the bend, he glances into the valley below: the town of Bourg d'Oisans glistening down there: the metal rooftops of houses; the Romanche River; the hoods of cars. Tiny from this height—colourful, bright items in a child's playset.

DMB's heart monitor bleeps: 158. Into the red zone. Seven kilometres per hour. He's barely moving. In this segment it takes forty seconds to cross one-tenth of each kilometre. Almost seven minutes to complete a kilometre.

This is hard work.

DMB has been bashed around in the past twenty-two months: five radioisotope treatments and most recently, in June, a liver surgery where they blocked up the arteries feeding the liver, in the hope of starving the larger tumours. Each treatment knocks him sideways for weeks. Recovery is slow. He does not fully overcome the fatigue before the next treatment knocks him on his body's door. It's the price to be paid for the possibility of holding off the disease's progress.

One pedal down; one pedal up.

On the tarmac they're passing over, the names of riders competing in the Tour de France are written in white paint: *Bauke, Laurens, Kittel.*

Virage #3. A young man wearing a white, yellow, and blue jersey pedals past. He's moving along at a clip, head bobbing, shoulders rolling. Some of the stretches between *virages* are more gentle than others. This is not one of them: 8.8 per cent. DMB grinds along. Head down. Pedal down; pedal up.

Here the words on the tarmac are stencilled in red, white, and blue: *team sky,* they read; *Froome dog.*

Two more young men in the blue, white, and yellow jerseys go past. They're working hard. Sweat runs down their noses and drips onto their bicycles.

A woman passes them on the straight stretch. She's hefty and sweating through her pink and black jersey. "*Bonjour,*" she gasps; "'*jour,*" DMB gasps back. No one is doing this climb easily.

Up ahead a man wearing an orange safety vest over his shirt is standing in the middle of the road taking photos of them as they approach: click click click. He hands them a business card as they pass: look up the photos on the Internet; if you like one, order it over the web.

Virage #1. As they go around, they pass the woman in pink and black. Her bicycle is wobbling; she's breathing heavily, drinking from her water bottle.

Last stretch. The road flattens here: only 3.5 per cent. Into the town of Huez. Past the bars with terraces occupied by cyclists, bikes propped along the deck railings. Kristen and DMB pull over. Sit for a moment on the edges of flowerpots in a parking lot. Here come two more of the boys from the yellow, blue, and white team. They hammer right to the finish.

Kristen takes his hand, squeezes it a moment. "I'm so proud of you," she says. "We did it," DMB says. Below their vantage point the boys from the team are taking off their jerseys and flapping them in the air. DMB can hardly believe he's made this climb. Most patients with carcinoid cancer consider a brisk two-kilometre walk an accomplishment. Many manage only a stroll around the block. He takes a couple of deep breaths. They take a few photos.

Now for the descent.

It's a lot to ask of a bicycle, that it sustain you through the blacks, build up your body, and strengthen your mind. Maybe it can do that. But can it keep you alive? It can build calf muscle and strengthen wrist bones, tighten abs and glutes, fortify your heart. It can lighten your days and lift your spirits. Maybe that's enough. You say to the handlebars, Hold me firm; you whisper to the pedals, Dance me round one more time; you implore the wheels, Keep up the momentum. Sustain me. You may say these things aloud sometimes: *save me*; on the shoulders of roads, head down, you get the strangest looks from joggers going the other way some mornings. Did you say the words aloud? You whisper them to your heart; that you know. Mostly you try not to think where it's all going, your puny existence on the planet, and in that way you're no different than anyone else: despite the death sentence you've been given, you don't dwell on death and dying, you try not to. How life punches you in the face; and how it winds down. It's defeatist; it's wallowing. There have been friends who have died—too soon, too soon—and friends who sit at the coffee shop with a grunt from arthritis or gasp when they walk to the car, from bronchial issues. Hospitals are not just where you go for procedures and treatments; they're also places where you sit at bedsides to comfort friends and family. Past the age of fifty, it's painful, all this death and dying—your parents, your aunts and uncles, your friends and colleagues and neighbours. To rise above the unbearable heaviness of being, some sing or dance or hammer on the piano until the fingertips drip blood. For me it's the bicycle, and it's a big burden to put on a simple machine with wheels. It's a lot to ask. But being proactive is important; it may be the key to well-being, if not survival. So when spirits are low and the day is dark, when it seems life is hardly worth going on with at all, jump on the saddle and ride out the blacks, without thinking, without anything but keeping those pedals in motion.

DEAD MAN ON A BIKE:

THE DEAD HAVE HAD THEIR SAY

I have achieved oneness with the road—now please dial 911 for me.
~ Unknown

Up on a ridge near Alma, Wisconsin. They've climbed from county road E up Blank Hill Road, a pleasant four-kilometre ascent at a not-too-demanding 4–6 per cent. Kristen can ride it at 20 k.p.h., but he's wary of the sacroiliac business, so he doesn't push past 15.

The ridge riding in this part of Wisconsin, Buffalo County, is lovely. The road is made of long, sweeping curves through corn and soy-bean fields, gentle undulations, with some sharpish ascents of several hundred metres, and some tight bends, a few at ninety degrees, gravel scattered over the tarmac by vehicles cutting through the apexes of curves, one tire in the shoulder.

The long descents push the computer over 40 k.p.h., the climbs drop it to 15. He enjoys taking the speed accumulated during descents into the next rise, jumping up to "attack" the hill in a high gear. Heart rate jumps to 150; mostly it hovers around 120.

The tarmac is smooth, few lumps and bumps, very few *road snakes*, rubbery repairs to cracks in asphalt surfaces that grab the rear wheel and can send you down for gravity tattoos. All the side roads in rural Wisconsin are near-perfect for cycling: terrific surfaces, exhilarating undulations, silence. Over the past eleven-kilometre stretch they've encountered three vehicles, two approaching, one passing, in something like a half hour. Otherwise, only the whirring of their own wheels.

They pull up at the Herold Cemetery, at the junction of two county roads. Inside the metal gate, there's a wooden gazebo with a bench where they sit and sip water. Look out over the tombstones, older ones tilting and sinking in the grass, more recent graves decked in flowers. Pervading silence. The dead have had their say.

He's brought a banana and he passes it to Kristen, who peels it and takes a bite. She passes it back, sips water. They're content with silence, the chirring of crickets, rustle of wind in nearby cornstalks. An unearthly silence; or rather, a quintessentially earthly silence, the hay bales exhaling their sweet odours, the soy leaves, cornstalks, roadside grasses. Silence like a drug. What is it Larkin says: we're reverential in churchyards, if only because "so many dead lie round"?

On these Wisconsin ridges you can see several kilometres in all directions: roads running to farmhouses, silver steel silos reflecting sun, red barns. "The prairies used to be like this," he says between bites of banana.

Kristen takes a sip of water. "How so?"

"Dotted with houses and outbuildings every kilometre or so. Now it's all these mega farms, abandoned houses, decaying barns."

"Agri-business."

"A shame."

"Things change."

"Got that right."

They sit in silence a while longer. He snaps several photos. They finish the banana, sip water.

"Time to go?"

"Yeah. Don't want the muscles to tighten up."

Back on the tarmac, then, sun hot on the neck, tires whirring, crows flapping across fields. Leave the dead to the dead.

Often when I head out on my bike—often but briefly—I wonder what my neighbours think as I pedal out of the bay we live in. I disappear down the road at 10:00 or 11:00 and don't return until 2:00 or 3:00. That's a long time to be out on a bike, turning pedals, fighting traffic, heart rate at an elevated level. One of my neighbours once said to me: riding that bike, it's a full-time job for you. Right. I haven't worked at an actual job for almost twenty years. Sometimes I make a joke about it: today I put a stamp on an envelope; tomorrow I plan on walking down to the mailbox and posting it. Plan on it. But I may not even get around to that. Of course I'm busy. I work on reviews and articles; edit other folks' manuscripts; write my books; post on my blog. These are all things I do at my own whim—and to my own schedule.

And ride my bike.

A host of things cross my mind while I'm out there, sails that drift onto the sea of my consciousness and then move off. I've been very lucky in my life: loved by wonderful women; privileged in my choice of vocation; serendipitous in my amazing son; blessed with intelligent and witty friends; fortunate in the way my finances have worked out: I've been independently wealthy for twenty years—if by that is meant that income exceeds expenses. Like most of my baby-boomer generation, I'm a fat cat (a fat cat who once "dissed" the system, one of the great ironies of our time, and, in particular, of my "flower-power" generation). My life has been wonderful.

It's also coming to an end. Terminal cancer is *terminal cancer.*

At the beginning of one of his books, the bastard with the yellow wristbands imagines how his own life will end: flashing down a mountain in Europe, his bike goes off the road, cartwheels crazily, throwing him off, tumbling over and over, until he comes to rest in a field of sunflowers, dead. I've imagined that death for myself: a sudden end while doing the thing I love, life leaking out of me as I gaze up at fluffy clouds and the wheels of my bike slow and finally cease spinning. Good-bye, world, it's been a great ride.

It's a wonderful fantasy: romantic, sentimental, and ultimately self-indulgent and foolish.

He knows, as I know, that to die going down a mountain road

you have to go off the tarmac a considerable distance from the bottom; you have to plunge down a ravine and land on outcroppings of rocks with enough force to split open your skull or break your spine. Otherwise, you might end up only badly hurt, a quadriplegic, or in a permanent coma, maimed but not defunct, eyes glazed over, hands twitching. Truly awful. Not to mention that landing on rocks and tree stumps in the final moments is a pretty grisly way to go: you might not die immediately, and instead of watching fluffy clouds you might be getting drenched as you twitch and slowly expire, like one of those squirrels on the side of the road.

And family? Suicide is a cruel punishment of family, who, even if prepared for this style of exit, willy-nilly, have a difficult time taking in your choice of the "Roman way out."

So, sorry, Tex, that ain't a-happenin'. We're enough of a pain in the ass to our families without suddenly saddling them with that final *coup d'egoisme.*

Years ago, when Kristen and I were riding the mountain bikes, we pedalled one afternoon past Poplar Point on Highway 26. It was a scorching day, and by the time we began the return journey, we'd gone almost fifty kilometres, and were looking at that again to get back to our neighbourhood in the south end of the city.

We struggled back to Nick's Inn, a landmark on the western limit of the city, and then pushed on toward the Perimeter Highway. But we were dehydrating at an alarming rate, and I was tiring fast. Sixty kilometres passed, seventy. It was stinking hot; at one point I'd poured water over my head to cool down. With more than twenty kilometres to go, we pulled over. We were both red-faced and about to drop over. "I'll call my dad," Kristen said.

I listened to a strained conversation, wishing we'd pushed on despite exhaustion. I don't like asking for help from anyone. *Be your own man,* my father was fond of saying: fierce independence bordering on psychosis. I see it in Andrew too. It's a family meme.

We were only a dozen kilometres from Kristen's parents' place near Headingley. When he pulled up in the pickup a few minutes later, Don was shaking his head. He'd never got the cycling thing. A golfer, he preferred "ruining a good walk," to quote Twain liberally. We put the bikes in the box of the pickup.

"Kristen," Don said as we pulled onto Roblin Boulevard on the way back into the city, "you can be a pain in the ass sometimes."

Kristen laughed and gave him a daughterly poke in the ribs.

I gritted my teeth and stared at the suburbs going by.

At home we threw off the bikes. I thanked Don again. "Bye, Dad," Kristen said, banging the pickup's door shut and laughing as we off-loaded the bikes.

He looked sheepish. "I didn't mean that," he called out in a trembling voice through his open window, "what I said back there."

"Yes, you did," Kristen said, still laughing. "But thanks anyway. We were dying out there. You saved us."

It was maybe literally true.

I think of that day often when I'm out on the bike. Isn't that what we do as parents? Rescue our loved ones? Isn't that what we do as children? We're a pain in the ass, every dumb-bunny one of us. We drop ourselves into shit and flounder about, arms and legs twitching, flailing. *Help.* And then love asserts itself. And we rescue someone—or are rescued by someone. It's the human journey, bicycle or no.

DEAD MAN ON A BIKE:

STORMY WEATHER

Is it splendid or stupid to take life seriously?
~ Gustave Flaubert

Starting at Larters at St. Andrews Golf Club north of Winnipeg, a road runs alongside the Red River in rolling landscape. Officially it's called Red River Drive, but there are several Red River drives in the area, so they call it the Lockport Ride. Twelve kilometres along the river.

They start on a Saturday morning in mixed sun and cloud, a north breeze in their faces, brisk but not cold. The forecasters have predicted the possibility of rain, 40 per cent chance, and both the sky and the heaviness of the air concur. Storms may be on the way. They're carrying—but not wearing—rain vests, *gilets*, the French call them, light but rain resistant.

It's a weekend in mid-September, the end of a hot and pleasant summer that has seen above-average temperatures most days, a terrific summer for cycling.

Seventy days have passed since the last radioisotope treatment, and Dead Man on a Bike is feeling close to 100 per cent. Though 100 per cent of what is a difficult question. Not, certainly, 100 per cent of what he would have felt like only ten years ago. Much of the time now, he's tired. When he gets the results of blood work, they're very low, below the low average range; many come back with little asterisk beside them: *nota bene!*

They pass Kennedy House, one of the grand houses along the route, converted now into a restaurant. They stop there for lunch sometimes, hearty soups, inventive sandwiches. A pleasant stop on a two- or three-hour ride.

A gentle ascent, then a sharpish climb. Here's Skinner's, a local favourite stop for hot dogs. Many cars parked outside, the pong of cooking meat. Then they pass the locks that give their name to the settlement. Swirling water on the other side, dozens of boats with anglers in them, fishing the waters.

The blood-work results are one indication that he's depleted. Run down. The other obvious one is the way he collapses on afternoons following two- and three-hour rides in the morning. Falls asleep watching TV while curled up on the sofa, Homer Simpson–style. The hope is that he'll recover strength now that the radio-therapies are over. Another is not scheduled until early 2013, leaving more than six months recovery time. Fingers crossed, then.

Overhead the sky is darkening, the sun nearly obliterated now. The north wind seems chillier here, though it may just be that here the wind is coming off the water. He glances at the sky: clouds that were fluffy an hour ago have become grey. Are they closer than before?

Just before they come to the junction with Highway 9 there's a dead critter on the side of the road. DMB feels a slight twinge in his gut. As they approach, he sees it's a ball of black and white fur, curled up, crumpled, the head hidden. Surprisingly, no flies are hovering about. Also surprisingly, the skunk does not smell. Are they sometimes hit before they have time to trigger their scent defence? It's logical. DMB will look that up when he gets home.

They wheel at Highway 9 and retrace their steps. It's their custom on these rides to do two laps, rather than extend the circuit north, as they've done numerous times in the past, through and then past the town of Selkirk.

On the return they encounter a lone cyclist outfitted in yellow jersey and shorts, yellow bike. Brief waves of greeting. Then there's a group of three men, heads down, doing a training ride. One of them is narrow and angular; his style of riding reminds him of a close friend who died in May after fighting various complications brought on by paraplegia. DMB takes in a shallow breath. A lump forms in his throat. They'd known each other since 1971, when they were young professors in Regina.

The leaves are dropping off the tree of life.

They'd taken trips together, DMB and his old pal, and their wives. Good trips, many laughs. The old boy loved wine and cheese, loved debating books and ideas, had a ready laugh and bright blue eyes. Then he fell one night in his own house and became an instant quadriplegic, confined for the remainder of his days to a wheelchair, six long and painful years.

DMB closes his eyes, takes in another shallow breath.

Yes, the sky is growing darker. But they may squeeze in another lap before the rain comes. He hopes they can.

One of my most recent memories is of lying on the couch in our TV room on a late afternoon. My heart was thumping at a high rate, I was having a bit of a struggle to breathe evenly. It was a hot late-summer day and I'd been out on a bike ride under clear skies beneath a blazing sun. I was pooped. A bottle of cool water was in one hand. I heard the back door open and close. Kristen arriving home from work. As a rule, I would have spent the past hour preparing supper, so that when she arrived we could spend an hour eating a meal, drinking wine, chatting amiably. Instead I was prone on the couch, dragged out.

When she came into the room, she said, "What happened?"

"Nothing, I was out on a bike ride."

She pursed her lips. She's a small, athletic woman. Her body speaks legends. "You rode fifty kilometres," she said flatly. "On a blazing hot day. When you're still recovering from the embolization."

"Yes."

"Why did you do that?" The statement was as much censure as observation.

I patted the couch. "Come here," I croaked. "Listen."

She sat down and took my hand. I shifted around into a half-sitting position.

"Listen," I began. "In the past years I've had to give up hockey. If I play on a Sunday morning with the Ice Mice, I'm exhausted, I spend the afternoon falling asleep watching football, chest aching, trying to regulate my breath. It's too hard on me. I can't do it any longer."

"And snoring."

We both laughed. "And snoring."

I paused. "When I go out on the bike I can no longer do the things I once did—ride a hundred kilometres, climb a serious hill, manage a pace over twenty-five kilometres per hour. The one thing I can still do, the one thing left to me, is ride fifty kilometres at a stretch. So I have to do that. You see? I have to."

"Even though . . ."

"Yeah. Even though."

She got up and went into the kitchen and came back with a washcloth soaked in cold water. She dabbed at my forehead. "You look awful."

"That feels good."

"Your cheeks are pale."

"It will pass," I croaked out.

"Yeah. Your heart rate will fall, the colour will return to your cheeks."

"I'll be alright."

She patted my leg with her free hand. "You're crazy," she said, "you're a crazy person, Wayne Tefs."

"Ain't we all."

"Ain't we all."

DEAD MAN ON A BIKE:

LAST BITE OF THE AVOCADO

You can't be sad while riding a bicycle.
~ Unknown

The first Saturday of December and the last in Tucson for the season, for the year 2013. It's warm as DMB and Kristen turn onto Catalina Highway heading toward the base of Mount Lemmon. They've debated whether or not to attempt the climb today and have decided not to, to avoid the risk of messing up his hips and back when they have the exhausting drive from Tucson to Phoenix ahead of them in the afternoon, and then the flight home to Winnipeg on Sunday. Better safe than sorry. Though it's a shame, too, on such a lovely day. Still, DMB is on the road and it's sunny and warm. (Back home on the frigid prairie the temperature is minus 4C and snowing.)

Lots of cyclists on the road. They pass a few: *mornin'/mornin'*. Cyclists approach from the opposite direction, having come off the mountain: nods, waves. Some hunched over handlebars, focused on making themselves as aerodynamic as possible. Bright jerseys, fully kitted out, swish bikes.

The road rises as it approaches Houghton, which cuts across it at ninety degrees. Up off the saddle. As they drop from the rise at Houghton and begin the last few kilometres to the foot of Mount Lemmon, the bikes pick up speed. Catalina Highway is lovely to ride: ample shoulder, smooth blacktop, just enough of a rise to challenge the legs.

There are houses set back from the highway on acreages, windbreaks of local shrubs, fences, gravel driveways. Suddenly to their right there's an open area and out of it are coming five javelinas, the desert pigs of the Tucson region. At some times of the year they're

dark grey in colour, but these are of a sandy tint, the largest leading the group, three babies following, another hefty beast to the
hindmost. They rear up at the approach of the cyclists, their black
snouts visible, the scruffy beards on the ends of their chins waver-
ing and trembling.

"Whoa," Kristen says. "Don't want to mess with those guys."

"Don't want to hurt them."

"Or more likely, be hurt by them."

It takes only a moment for Kristen and DMB to pass the beasts.
Though they slowed, the javelinas have moved toward the shoulder and must be poised to cross behind them. Kristen does a quick
shoulder check. "They're on the road now," she reports, "they're
okay, the cars are stopping." DMB feels a warm wave rush through
his chest and into his bowels. He lets a long breath out of his nose.
A cyclist coming towards them points towards the javelinas, and
they wave back: *we know, we know.*

"Huge," DMB says in a moment. "Was that the mother up
front?"

"The sow," Kristen says. "And the male in the rear. They look so
stocky and solid."

"And wild."

"Yes. No knowing what they might do. But aren't they night
creatures?"

"Supposed to be. But that family I saw in the spring were out
around noon."

"Yeah, I remember."

Neat, they agree. Though probably the residents in the area
aren't so keen. Javelinas can destroy a vegetable garden in a few
minutes. And they're not creatures to mess with: they charge at
human beings, they bite, they kick.

They ride on in silence, thinking of what they've just seen. In
a kilometre they notice the pull of the uphill as the climb proper
approaches. DMB gears down: out of the big ring. Trying to maintain a spin at over 80 rpm.

"Do you hear it?" he asks.

Kristen gives him a quizzical look.

"The siren song of Mount Lemmon," he says, grinning. "*Kristen, Kristen.* The climb is calling to you."

She laughs. "I hear it, yes."

"Plug your ears with wax."

"Like the Argonauts had to do."

They laugh. The climb does call out, as do all challenges of its kind: put yourself to the test now, come on now, go for it, see what you're made of. All athletes and all jocks know the seductive call of the physical trial. Those songs are what they live by—and die by, too. As they swing right at Soldier Trail, Kristen looks up the road to the mountain and sighs. "Another day," she says.

"Next year," DMB says. "Spring is just weeks away."

It does not matter how slowly you go … So long as you do not stop
~ Confucius

DEAD MAN ON A BIKE:

IT'S ALL GOOD, IT'S ALL OK.

He's pedalling the bike in Tucson, Arizona, a bright and sunny April morning with a gentle breeze from the south on his left cheek. It's hot, 80F, the weather gal says just as he's preparing to start this ride, going to 90F—what's that in *new money*, he wonders—30C? Hot. Hot in the hills of Tucson.

Cars pass, pickup trucks, a school bus on its way to begin its route. He checks his watch: 7:30. They start school early in the desert. Pickups whizz by, many dragging wagons behind with rakes and shovels attached to wire mesh walls; there's a lot of yard clean-up work in Tucson. It's surrounded by desert, but there's lots of greenery around. The wagons rattle as they bounce by on the tarmac. Elbows project from the truck windows, cigarettes dangling from tanned fingers, start of a workday. Springtime in the desert; and springtime in his heart, too. While riding a bicycle, he's learned, metaphors abound: turn a corner and your wheels bump over one.

Birds twitter in the bushes along the roadside, doves coo from rooftops. A crow sitting on the top of a telephone pole barks at him as he pedals past. "I salute you, crow," he calls out and laughs to himself. He's the dead man on a bike.

Cars whizz by, but they're no issue for cyclists. In Tucson there are dedicated bike lanes on almost every street, *real* bike lanes, he thinks, most three feet wide and many five and seven feet wide. And motorists respect them—and the cyclists in them. Tucson is a cycling haven. It has been named one of the best places in the USA for road cycling. Portland for commuters, Tucson for roadies.

He's coming up to an intersection controlled by lights and takes a slug from his water bottle. The three kilometres he's just put behind him have been flat, flattish, a gentle climb, *false flat,* cyclists say, but up ahead looms a steep and sharp climb, not long, which is followed by a descent, then another steeper climb, and so on. It's the Catalina Foothills.

He waits for the light to turn, takes another slug from the bottle. Ready, he says to himself, ready for those hills. He's the dead man on a bike. He's been the dead man on a bike for nineteen years, going on twenty. He's the dead man on a bike but it's all good, it's all okay.